Get Through MRCPsych CASC

Get Through MRCPsych CASC, Second Edition, is intended for psychiatric trainees sitting the CASC component of the MRCPsych exam. Written by authors with long-term expertise in the field, the text provides over 100 stations closely matched to the subjects that appear in the actual exam, along with concise synopses, helpful tables of categories of enquiry and specimen enquiries, and common pitfalls.

Melvyn Zhang Weibin, MBBS (Singapore), DCP (Ireland), MRCPsych (United Kingdom), FAMS (Singapore): Assistant Professor, Lee Kong Chian School of Medicine, Nanyang Technological University, Singapore, and Consultant Psychiatrist, National Addictions Management Service, Institute of Mental Health, Singapore.

Cyrus Ho Su Hui, MBBS (Singapore), Dip (Cl Psy) (RCP&S, Ireland), MRCPsych (United Kingdom), Grad Dip Acupuncture (Singapore), MSc (Research) (Singapore), MSc (Applied Neuroscience) (United Kingdom), PhD (Singapore), FAMS (Psych) (Singapore), IFAPA (United States of America): Assistant Professor and Consultant Psychiatrist and Director, Psychiatry Undergraduate Education, National University of Singapore and National University Hospital, Singapore.

Roger Ho, MBBS (Hong Kong), MD (Hong Kong), DPM (Ireland), DCP (Ireland), GDip in Psychotherapy (Singapore), MMed (Psych) (Singapore), MCPsychI (Ireland), FRCPsych (United Kingdom), FRCP (Canada), FRCP (Edinburgh), FAMS (Psych): Professor and Senior Consultant Psychiatrist at the Department of Psychological Medicine, National University of Singapore, and National University Hospital, Singapore.

Basant K. Puri, MA, PhD, MB, BChir, MSc, MMath, FRCPsych, FRMS, FRSB: C.A.R., Cambridge, and University of Winchester, United Kingdom.

GET THROUGH

About the Series

Our bestselling *Get Through* series guides medical postgraduates through the many exams they will need to pass throughout their career, whatever their specialty. Each title is written by authors with recent first-hand experience of the exam, overseen and edited by experts in the field to ensure each question or scenario closely matches the latest examining board guidelines. Detailed explanations and background knowledge provide all you need to know to get through your postgraduate medical examination.

Get Through MRCOG Part 1
2E
Rekha Wuntakal, Ziena Abdullah, and Tony Hollingworth

Get Through MRCOG Part 2
EMQs
Kalaivani Ramalingam, Latha Mageswari Palanivelu, Lakshmi Thirumalaikumar

Get Through MRCOG Part 3
Clinical Assessment 2E
T Justin Clark, Arri Coomarasamy, Justin Chu and Paul Smith

Get Through MRCOG Part 2
SBAs
Rekha Wuntakal, Madhavi Kalindindi and Tony Hollingworth

Get Through Final FRCR 2A
SBAs
Teck Yew Chin, Susan Cheng Shelmerdine, Akash Ganguly and Chinedum Anoksike

Get Through MRCPsych Paper A1
Mock Examination Papers
Melvyn WB Zheng, Cyrus SH Ho, Roger Ho, Ian H Treasaden and Basant K Puri

Get Through MRCPsych CASC
Melvyn WB Zheng, Cyrus SH Ho, Roger Ho, Ian H Treasaden and Basant K Puri

Get Through MRCS Part A
SBAs
Nikhil Pawa, Paul Cathcart and Howard Tribe

Get Through DRCOG
SBAs, EMQs and McQs
Rekha Wuntakal, Madhavi Kalidindi and Tony Hollingworth

For more information about this series please visit: *www.crcpress.com/ Get-Through/book-series/CRCGETTHROUG*

Get Through MRCPsych CASC

Second Edition

Melvyn Zhang Weibin, Cyrus Ho Su Hui,
Roger Ho and Basant K. Puri

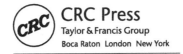

CRC Press
Taylor & Francis Group
Boca Raton London New York

CRC Press is an imprint of the
Taylor & Francis Group, an **informa** business

Second edition published 2024
by CRC Press
6000 Broken Sound Parkway NW, Suite 300, Boca Raton, FL 33487–2742

and by CRC Press
4 Park Square, Milton Park, Abingdon, Oxon, OX14 4RN

CRC Press is an imprint of Taylor & Francis Group, LLC

© 2024 Melvyn Zhang Weibin, Cyrus Ho Su Hui, Roger Ho, Basant K. Puri

This book contains information obtained from authentic and highly regarded sources. While all reasonable efforts have been made to publish reliable data and information, neither the author[s] nor the publisher can accept any legal responsibility or liability for any errors or omissions that may be made. The publishers wish to make clear that any views or opinions expressed in this book by individual editors, authors or contributors are personal to them and do not necessarily reflect the views/opinions of the publishers. The information or guidance contained in this book is intended for use by medical, scientific or health-care professionals and is provided strictly as a supplement to the medical or other professional's own judgement, their knowledge of the patient's medical history, relevant manufacturer's instructions and the appropriate best practice guidelines. Because of the rapid advances in medical science, any information or advice on dosages, procedures or diagnoses should be independently verified. The reader is strongly urged to consult the relevant national drug formulary and the drug companies' and device or material manufacturers' printed instructions, and their websites, before administering or utilizing any of the drugs, devices or materials mentioned in this book. This book does not indicate whether a particular treatment is appropriate or suitable for a particular individual. Ultimately it is the sole responsibility of the medical professional to make his or her own professional judgements, so as to advise and treat patients appropriately. The authors and publishers have also attempted to trace the copyright holders of all material reproduced in this publication and apologize to copyright holders if permission to publish in this form has not been obtained. If any copyright material has not been acknowledged please write and let us know so we may rectify in any future reprint.

ISBN: 978-1-032-32156-1 (hbk)
ISBN: 978-1-032-32154-7 (pbk)
ISBN: 978-1-003-31311-3 (ebk)

DOI: 10.1201/9781003313113

Typeset in Minion
by Apex CoVantage, LLC

CONTENTS

Topic II   Geriatric psychiatry

Topic III   Child psychiatry

Topic IV Learning disabilities

Topic V Addictions and substance misuse

Topic VI Psychotherapies

Topic VII Eating disorders

Topic VIII Personality disorder

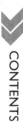

CONTENTS

PREFACE

This book consists of over 100 stations for the Royal College of Psychiatrists Clinical Assessment of Skills and Competencies (CASC) examination. This book has been updated, and the stations have been redesigned to reflect the style and types of stations that are commonly encountered in the MRCPsych examination at the time of this writing. This book has also been reformatted, such that it is in-line with the new CASC exam guidelines.

While conventional CASC revision materials provide trainees with only a short description of the task required in each station and the key points to cover, or communication skills required, this book differentiates itself from other revision materials. In each of the stations covered, we provide trainees with additional information such as an outline of the station and a CASC grid with suggested questions to ask in each of the stations. In addition, we have provided some of the common issues that might result in trainees not meeting the requirements for a passing grade in the station.

We welcome any feedback from our readers. We wish to thank all our past readers for your comments and all the authors who contributed to this revision guidebook.

AUTHOR BIOGRAPHIES

Melvyn Zhang Weibin: MBBS (Singapore), DCP (Ireland), MRCPsych (United Kingdom), FAMS (Singapore).

Assistant Professor Melvyn Zhang currently works as Assistant Professor and Consultant, Psychiatrist at the Lee Kong Chian School of Medicine, Nanyang Technological University and the National Addictions Management Service, Institute of Mental Health, Singapore. He graduated with his basic medical degree from the National University of Singapore in 2011 and obtained his diploma in clinical psychiatry from the Royal of Physicians and Surgeons, Ireland, in 2014. He obtained his membership with the Royal College of Psychiatrists in 2014. In 2016, he completed his residency training in psychiatry in Singapore and joined the National Addictions Management Service at the Institute of Mental Health. In 2016, he also obtained his fellowship with the Academy of Medicine, Singapore. His clinical interests are in the treatment of individuals with addictive disorders, and his special interest is in treating adolescents with Internet gaming disorder. Professor Zhang has published over 120 papers in peer reviewed papers. He is also currently serving on the editorial boards of the *British Journal of Psychiatry (BJPsych), Journal of Internet Medical Research (JMIR), Mental Health and Technology* and *Healthcare*. He is also very involved in medical education and has been teaching medical students from the National University of Singapore and the Lee Kong Chian School of Medicine, Nanyang Technological University.

Cyrus Ho Su Hui: MBBS (Singapore), Dip (Cl Psych) (RCP&S, Ireland), MRCPsych (United Kingdom), Grad Dip Acupuncture (Singapore), MSc (Research) (Singapore), MSc (Applied Neuroscience) (United Kingdom), PhD (Singapore), FAMS (Psych) (Singapore), IFAPA (United States of America).

Assistant Professor Cyrus Ho Su Hui is General Adult and Consultation Liaison Psychiatrist managing psychiatric conditions across the age continuum from adolescence to old age, with special interest interfacing between medicine and psychiatry, complex mood disorders, and neuropsychiatry. After graduating with a bachelor of medicine and bachelor of surgery (MBBS) from the National University of Singapore (NUS), Dr Ho obtained a diploma in clinical psychiatry from Ireland. He was conferred memberships to the Royal College of Psychiatrists from the United Kingdom and College of Psychiatrists of Ireland. He is a fellow of the Singapore Academy of Medicine, and he received the International Fellowship to the American Psychiatric Association. With a keen interest in neuroscience, he earned a master of science in research from NUS for his research work on neuroimaging in depressed and chronic pain patients. He was further awarded distinction in the master of science in applied neuroscience from King's College London. His PhD dissertation was on integrating multimodal biomarkers to aid the diagnosis and treatment of major depressive disorder. Under the MOH Health Manpower Development Plan (HMDP) award, he underwent further training in neuropsychiatry with Montreal Neurological Hospital in Canada and Royal Melbourne Neuropsychiatry Unit in Australia. Being an avid researcher, Dr Ho has extensively published more than 300 academic papers in international peer-reviewed journals, including *The Lancet, Annals of Internal Medicine, Autoimmunity Reviews, EBioMedicine*, and *Brain, Behavior, and Immunity*. He frequently delivers presentations in international psychiatry conferences, including notable ones such as the American Psychiatric Association (APA) Annual Meeting and the European Congress of Psychiatry. Dr Ho is a passionate educator involved in teaching both students and residents alike. He currently serves as NUS Psychiatry Undergraduate Education Director. His dedication in education is exemplified by various teaching awards, such as the Dean's Award for Teaching Excellence in 2015, 2016, 2018, 2020, and 2021 and Junior Doctor Teaching Award in 2015. He co-authored four postgraduate guidebooks for residents published by Taylor and Francis and an undergraduate textbook titled *Mastering Psychiatry*, which is a popular reference book used by local medical students.

Roger Ho: MBBS (Hong Kong), MD (Hong Kong), DPM (Ireland), DCP (Ireland), GDip in Psychotherapy (Singapore), MMed (Psych) (Singapore), MCPsychI (Ireland), FRCPsych (United Kingdom), FRCP (Canada), FRCP (Edinburgh), FAMS (Psych).

Professor Ho currently works as Professor and Senior Consultant Psychiatrist at the Department of Psychological Medicine, National University of Singapore (NUS) and National University Hospital (NUH). He is Research Director coordinating research studies for the department. He is also Principal Investigator and Director of the functional near infrared spectroscopy (fNIRS) lab at the Institute for Health Innovation and Technology (iHealthtech, NUS).

Professor Ho joined the Department of Psychological Medicine, NUH, in July 2002 as a medical officer. Professor Ho did his psychiatry residency and fellowship training at the Department of Psychological Medicine, NUH, and rose through the academic and clinical ranks in NUS and NUH.

Professor Ho obtained his basic medical degree (MBBS) from the University of Hong Kong. He received the master of medicine (MMED) in psychiatry from the National University of Singapore. He received his higher research degree, doctor of medicine by research (MD), from the University of Hong Kong.

He is a fellow of the Royal College of Psychiatrists (UK), Royal College of Physicians (Canada), Royal College of Physicians (Edinburgh) and Academy of Medicine (Singapore).

Professor Ho has clinical and research interests in applying functional near infrared spectroscopy (fNIRS) in diagnosing psychiatric disorders, including attention deficit and hyperactivity disorder (ADHD), borderline personality disorder, major depressive disorder, and dementia. He has conducted research to improve the accuracy of psychiatric diagnosis by machine learning and has translated his research findings into clinical implementations at NUS iHealthtech.

Professor Ho is involved in multiple research endeavours, which primarily aim to study the interface between psychiatry and medicine. His earlier research involves elucidating psychiatric symptoms associated with medical disorders, including systemic lupus erythematosus, diabetes, and eczema, as well as medical complications of depression and buprenorphine misuse. His research extended to the laboratory and the study of effects of antidepressants on the immune system in animals. During the COVID-19 pandemic, he conducted global mental health research to study the psychological impact of the pandemic in different countries.

Professor Ho has published over 500 papers in peer reviewed journals (H-index > 77). In 2021, he was identified by Clarivate Analytics (Web of Science) as one of the Most Highly Cited and Influential Researchers in the world. Professor Ho is extensively involved in medical education. He disseminated psychiatric knowledge through publications of academic books with global influence. An example is the co-authorship and publication of a postgraduate textbook, *Revision Notes in Psychiatry (3rd edition)*, CRC Press, and this book has been one of the most commonly used reference texts since 1998 by psychiatric trainees in Commonwealth countries. Professor Ho has received numerous awards throughout his academic career, including the NUS Annal Teaching Excellence Award in 2012 and Special Recognition Award (2016–2020). He has supervised many medical students through the Undergraduate Research Opportunity Programme (UROP) and been main/co-supervisor for more than 20 MSc/PhD candidates. He is a regular PhD qualifying examination and oral defence examiner for other departments and faculties at NUS.

Basant K. Puri: MA, PhD, MB, BChir, MSc, MMath, FRCPsych, FRMS, FRSB.

Professor Puri is based at C.A.R., Cambridge, and the University of Winchester, UK. He has authored or co-authored several books, including *Drugs in Psychiatry*, *Textbook of Psychiatry*, and *Clinical Neuropsychiatry and Neuroscience Fundamentals*.

TOPIC I
GENERAL ADULT PSYCHIATRY

STATION 1
OBSESSIVE-COMPULSIVE
DISORDER

Information to candidates:

Name of patient: Mr Lopez

Mr Lopez has been referred by his GP to the mental health service for excessive hand washing.

Task: Please speak to Mr Lopez and obtain a detailed history to arrive at a diagnosis. Please also rule out other comorbidity.

Outline of station:

You are Mr Lopez, and you have been having increased fears of contamination ever since a laboratory accident that happened six months ago, where there was a chemical leakage. Ever since then, you realized that, due to your constant fears, you always needed to wash your hands multiple times to reduce the fears. This has affected your life significantly as you are always late for appointments, and you are contemplating quitting your job at the lab.

CASC Construct Table:

The CASC Construct Table is formatted such that candidates would be able to cover adequately both the range and depth of the assessment required in this station.

Starting off: "Hello, I am Dr Melvyn. I have received some information from your GP regarding the difficulties that you have been having. Would you mind telling me more?"			
Core OCD symptoms	Origin of thoughts	Exploration of other obsessional thoughts	Exploration of other compulsions
	Can you tell me more about those worries that you have been having? How long have you have had them? Do those thoughts come from within your mind, or are they imposed by outside persons or influences?	Are you also concerned about needing to arrange things in a special way? Do you also have thoughts, images, or doubts that keep coming to your mind?	Do you find yourself needing to check very frequently? Do you find yourself needing to perform other rituals to prevent something bad from happening?

DOI: 10.1201/9781003313113-1

	Nature of thoughts Are those thoughts that you have repetitive in nature? Are they bothering you consistently even though you do not wish to have them?	Exploration of compulsions Tell me more about how you have been dealing with those obsessional thoughts? How do you feel after performing the rituals?	When did your symptoms start? Assess circumstances of the onset of symptoms and progression (any worsening?)
Current functioning	Impact of illness Could you tell me how these rituals have impacted your life?	Have they affected other areas of your life, such as your relationships?	Any medical complications from your symptoms? For example, dermatological problems from excessive handwashing? (Please offer to check the skin if the patient has this problem.)
Other symptoms	Assessment for depressive symptoms How has your mood been? Are you still interested in things you used to enjoy?	How have you been sleeping? How has your appetite been? Have these mood symptoms come on before your OCD symptoms?	Are there other worries that you have been having?
Coping mechanisms	It has been a difficult time for you. Have you used alcohol to help you get through these difficult times?	Have you used any other drugs to help you cope with this challenging time?	

Common pitfalls:

a. Failure to cover the range and depth of the OCD symptoms.
b. Failure to assess the impact of the symptoms.

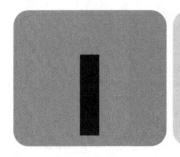

Information to candidates:

Name of patient: Mr Smith

Mr Smith has been brought into the hospital for an assessment today as he went to the police, telling them that he is surrendering for a terrible crime that he has committed. The medics have done basic blood and radiological investigations, which were all normal. However, they have called you, the psychiatric trainee on call, to request that you assess him.

Task: Perform a mental state examination, looking for any delusional beliefs and any other psychopathology that he has.

Outline of station:

You are Mr Smith, a 45-year-old postman. You have surrendered yourself to the police today as you firmly believe that you are responsible for a war between Iraq and Russia. You are extremely guilty for causing the war as you feel that it is all because of a silly mistake which you made three months ago whilst sorting out the mail in the Royal Mail headquarters. It troubles you much when you see or hear of the death toll from the war. You decide to surrender yourself today as the police have been commenting and telling you that you should. Your mood is terrible, and you have been having poor sleep as the police keep speaking to you. You are terrified whenever you see a white car as you believe that it might be the police who are monitoring your every move. You have had passive suicidal ideations but have not made any suicide plans. On seeing the doctor, you request and demand that he gives you an injection immediately, as you feel it might be better off dead than to feel guilty constantly. You will appear distracted and preoccupied at times. When asked, tell the candidate that the police are around and speak directly to you.

CASC Construct Table:

The CASC Construct Table is formatted such that candidates would be able to cover adequately both the range and depth of the assessment required in this station.

DOI: 10.1201/9781003313113-2

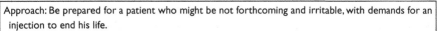

Approach: Be prepared for a patient who might be not forthcoming and irritable, with demands for an injection to end his life. Starting off: "Hello, I am Dr Melvyn, one of the psychiatrists from the mental health unit. I understand that the police brought you here today. Can you tell me more?" If the patient is difficult: "It seems to me that you are quite distressed. I'm here to help you. Can you tell me more about why you're here today?"			
Elicit delusional beliefs and challenging the belief	Can you tell me more as to why you feel this way?	Do you feel that you are guilty and responsible for all that has happened? Assess the degree of conviction: How convinced are you: totally or partially? How did you arrive at this conclusion?	Could there be any other alternative explanations for this? Could it be because there are long-standing political tensions between the two countries? **Nihilistic delusions** You mentioned that you'd be better off dead? Could you tell me more? Do you feel that you're already dead?
Elicit depressive symptoms	With all these ongoing, how has your mood been? Are you able to enjoy the things that you used to enjoy?	How has your sleep been? Have there been any problems with your appetite? How have your energy levels been?	
Risk assessment	Have you had thoughts of ending your life previously?	Do you still have thoughts of ending your life right now?	What plans do you have in mind? Is there anything that will prevent you from doing so?
Elicit hallucinations	**Auditory hallucinations** Do you hear sounds or voices that others do not hear? How many voices can you hear? Are they as clear as our current conversation?	**Second-person auditory hallucinations** Do they speak to you? Can you give me examples of what they have been saying to you?	**Third-person auditory hallucinations** Do they refer to you as "he" or "she"? Do they comment on your actions? Do they give you orders or commands as to what to do? How do you feel when you hear them? Could there be any alternative explanations for these experiences that you have been having? Assess for other modalities of hallucinations: visual, gustatory, olfactory, and tactile.

(Continued)

(Continued)

Elicit thought disorders	Thought interference Do you feel that your thoughts are being interfered with? Who do you think is doing this?	Thought insertion Do you have thoughts in your head you feel are not your own? Where do you think these thoughts come from?	Thought broadcasting and insertion Do you feel that your thoughts are being broadcasted such that others know what you are thinking? **Thought withdrawal** Do you feel that your thoughts are being taken away from your head by some external forces?
Elicit passivity experiences	Do you feel in control of your own actions and emotions?	Do you feel that someone or something is trying to control you?	Who or what do you think this would be?

Common pitfalls:

a. Failure to take control of the interview/inadequate knowledge of how to handle a difficult patient.
b. Failure to challenge the core delusion adequately.
c. Failure to elicit other delusional beliefs and cover the range and depth of other perceptual abnormalities.
d. Failure to perform a risk assessment.
e. Failure to assess for depressive symptoms and wrongly concluding that the patient has schizophrenia.
f. Failure to conclude and demonstrate to the examiner that the patient has a strong sense of guilt arising from severe depression.

STATION 3
OUTPATIENT MSE
REVIEW

Information to candidates:

Name of patient: Mr Donoghue

Mr Donoghue has been known to the mental health service since age 20. He has been previously diagnosed with schizophrenia and has had multiple previous admissions. He is here today for his routine outpatient review.

Task: Assess first-rank symptoms and specific symptomatology.

Outline of station:

You are Mr Donoghue, and you have had schizophrenia since you were 20 years old. You used to have multiple admissions to the mental health service, mostly under section. Your relapses were common due to your non-compliance with medication. In the past two years, you have been more regular with your medication as you now have a community psychiatric nurse supervising you and your medication. You have been compliant with your medication ever since then. You are here today for your routine review. You will report to the psychiatrist that you have been feeling increasingly anxious recently. You do not have all the symptoms typical of an anxiety disorder. Late into the interview, disclose to the psychiatrist that you have been feeling increasingly anxious as you could hear the neighbours making demeaning remarks about you having schizophrenia. You hear them commenting loudly near the wall next to their house. You do not have any other first rank symptoms. You do not use any alcohol or substance.

CASC Construct Table:

The CASC Construct Table is formatted such that candidates would be able adequately to cover both the range and depth of the assessment required in this station.

DOI: 10.1201/9781003313113-3

Approach: Be prepared for a patient who might minimize all the psychotic symptoms. Demonstration of empathy is crucial towards eliciting symptomatology.
Starting off: "Hello, I am Dr Melvyn, one of the psychiatrists from the mental health unit. I understand that you are here today for your routine appointment."
"Could you tell me how you've been?"

Eliciting auditory hallucinations	Auditory hallucinations Do you hear sounds or voices that others do not hear? How many voices could you hear? Are they as clear as our current conversation? What do they say?	Second-person auditory hallucinations Do they speak directly to you? Can you give me some examples of what they have been saying to you?	Third-person auditory hallucinations Do they refer to you as "he" or "she," much like a third person? Do they comment on your actions? Do they give you orders or commands as to what to do?	How do you feel when you hear them? Could there be any alternative explanation for these experiences that you have been having?
Eliciting hallucinations in all other modalities	Olfactory Recently, has there been anything wrong with your smell? Can you tell me more about it?	Gustatory Have you noticed that the food or drink seemed to have a different taste recently?	Somatic Have you had any strange feelings in your body?	Visual Have you been able to see things that other people can't see? What kind of things could you see? Could you give me an example? How long has this been for?
Elicit thought disorders	Thought interference Do you feel that your thoughts are being interfered with? Who do you think is doing this?	Thought insertion Do you have thoughts in your head that you feel are not your own? Where do you think these thoughts come from?	Thought broadcasting Do you feel that your thoughts are being broadcasted such that others would know what you are thinking?	Thought withdrawal Do you feel that your thoughts are being taken away from your head by some external force?
Elicit passivity experiences	Do you feel in control of your own actions and emotions?	Do you feel that someone or something is trying to control you? Who or what do you think this would be?		

Impact of symptoms on mood and coping mechanisms	I understand that this must be a difficult time for you. How have you been coping?	Has this affected your mood in any way? Are you still interested in the things you used to enjoy? Are there any difficulties with your sleep or appetite?	Have you made use of any substances, such as alcohol, to help you cope? What about street drugs?	
Risk assessment— risk to self and others	Are you feeling so troubled that you have entertained thoughts of ending your life? What plans have you made?	Have you made any plans to confront your neighbours?		

Common pitfalls:

a. Failure to cover the range and depth of information.
b. Failure to engage the patient (who is minimizing his symptoms to avoid being sectioned) and elicit the core information.
c. Failure to assess for all core first-rank symptoms (auditory hallucinations, three types of thought interference, control of mood, movement, intention by external agents, and other delusions).
d. Poor time management.

STATION 4
MANIA WITH
PSYCHOTIC SYMPTOMS

Information to candidates:

Name of patient: Ms Green

Ms Green has been brought into the hospital for an assessment today. She was caught speeding down the M1 motorway at more than 90 miles per hour. When the police arrested her, her mood was noted to be irritable. The medical doctor has seen her and has done the routine lab work, to which nothing abnormal has been found. The medical doctor has given her oral lorazepam to calm her down. She is slightly less irritable now and is more willing to speak to the psychiatrist.

Task: Perform a mental state examination, looking for any abnormal psychopathologies that may be suggestive of mania with psychotic symptoms

Outline of station:

You are Ms Green, a 29-year-old female. You have been arrested by the police for speeding down the M1 motorway at more than 90 miles per hour. Your mood has been high for the past week or so. You believe that the royal family has granted you special rights and powers, and hence you are confident that you will not get into any forensic trouble if you speed. You are irritated that the police have brought you into the hospital for an assessment for no reason. You share with the doctor that you are the chosen one of the royal family. You are absolutely convinced about this. You have special rights and abilities that others do not have. You have not been sleeping well due to the increasing number of thoughts that you have. At times, you feel that you could hear the royal family speaking directly to you. Apart from speeding, you have donated £3,000 over the past week to a local charity.

CASC Construct Table:

The CASC Construct Table is formatted such that candidates would be able adequately to cover both the range and depth of the assessment required in this station.

DOI: 10.1201/9781003313113-4

Approach: Be prepared to expect a patient with florid manic symptoms who might be difficult to engage. Be prepared that the patient might be disinhibited—setting boundaries is crucial, and be prepared to call for a chaperone.

Starting off: "Hello, I am Dr Melvyn, one of the psychiatrists from the mental health unit. I understand that the police brought you here today. Could you tell me more?"

Eliciting core manic symptoms	How have you been feeling in your mood? If I were to ask you to rate your mood on a scale from 1 to 10, what score would you give your mood now? Have others commented that you have been more irritable recently?	How has your energy level been? How has your sleep been? Are you still as energetic as ever despite the decreased amount of sleep? How has your appetite been?	Are you able to think clearly? Do you feel that there are many thoughts racing through your mind at any moment?	How long have you been feeling this way?
Eliciting grandiose delusional beliefs and challenging beliefs	It seems to me that you feel that you are specially chosen. Could you tell me more?	Are there any special powers or abilities that you have that others do not have? Could you tell me more about it?	Could there be any other explanations for why you are having all these symptoms/all these special abilities? Could it be because you have been unwell?	Do you feel increasingly more confident about yourself recently?
Eliciting hallucinations in all other modalities, eliciting thought disorders, eliciting passivity experiences	Auditory hallucinations Do you hear sounds or voices that others do not hear? How many voices could you hear? Are they as clear as our current conversation? What do they say?	Second-person auditory hallucinations Do they speak directly to you? Can you give me some examples of what they have been saying to you?	Third-person auditory hallucinations Do they refer to you as "he" or "she," much like a third person? Do they comment on your actions? Do they give you orders or commands as to what to do?	How do you feel when you hear them? Could there be any alternative explanation for these experiences that you have been having? Do you feel that your thoughts are being interfered with by an external force? Do you feel in control of your own actions and emotions?

(Continued)

(Continued)

Risk assessment—risk of excessive spending, intimacy, self-harm, violence	Have you engaged in any activities recently that might be dangerous? By that, I mean, have you been involved with the police recently?	Have you been spending more money than usual?	Have you been recently involved in any intimate relationships with others?	Have you been so troubled by all these that you have entertained thoughts of ending your life? Have you got into trouble with others around you?
Impact and coping mechanisms	How have you been coping with all these?	Have you made use of any substances, such as alcohol, to help you cope?	What about street drugs?	
Previous psychiatric history	Have you received any help/assistance from any mental health professionals?	Have you been diagnosed with depression before?	Have you been on a course of antidepressants? Are you still consuming them now?	

It would be helpful to use reflective interview techniques in this case to demonstrate the symptoms portrayed by the patient. For example, "I can see that you are talking very fast now. I'm wondering if your thoughts are racing just as fast?" "You are talking fast and seem to have a lot of energy. Am I right? I'm wondering how your sleep has been?" In these two illustrations, one can link up and cluster symptoms together to make the flow of the interview more seamless and logical.

Common pitfalls:

a. Failure to take control of the station.
b. Failure to set boundaries with patient.
c. Failure to elicit core manic symptoms from patient/failure to cover the range and depth of the station.
d. Failure to perform a complete risk assessment.
e. Failure to assess for depressive symptoms and recent use of antidepressants that may precipitate mania.

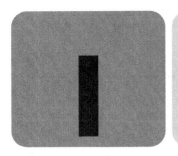

STATION 5
HYPOMANIA

Information to candidates:

Name of patient: Mr Brown

Mr Brown has been referred by his GP for an assessment with the local mental health service. He has been diagnosed with depressive disorder since the age of 18 years old and has been treated with several antidepressants, including that of fluoxetine, sertraline, and most recently, venlafaxine. He was started on venlafaxine: he did not respond well to the previous trials of antidepressants as his energy levels were markedly low. Since the commencement of venlafaxine for the past week, his energy has markedly improved. He has been describing that he has been experiencing feelings of elation, with occasional racing thoughts. You have been asked to speak to him to perform a mental state examination.

Task: Perform a mental state examination, looking for abnormal psychopathologies that may suggest a hypomania episode.

Outline of station:

You are Mr Brown, a 30-year-old male. You have been on regular follow-ups with your GP for depression. You have tried two different SSRIs (fluoxetine and sertraline), but they did not help alleviate your mood symptoms. Your energy remained persistently low, making it hard to function at work. You have been performing poorly at your work, which involves real estate investments. Since the switch of the antidepressant over to venlafaxine, your mood has been subjectively better. Over the last four days, you have been feeling elated. You realize that you now require less sleep (three to four hours is sufficient), and your energy remains good. You feel that you're better able to handle your work. You have been spending more, buying personal items like clothes, as you feel that personal grooming is important. You have at times had racing thoughts of wanting to take trips overseas, to meet new clients, and to share with them new investment opportunities. You have not been experiencing any abnormal perceptions.

CASC Construct Table:

The CASC Construct Table is formatted such that candidates would be able adequately to cover both the range and depth of the assessment required in this station.

DOI: 10.1201/9781003313113-5

Approach: Be prepared that the patient might be disinhibited—setting boundaries is crucial, and be prepared to call for a chaperone. Starting off: "Hello, I am Dr Melvyn, one of the psychiatrists from the mental health unit. I understand that your local GP has referred you here today. Could you tell me more?"				
Eliciting core hypomanic symptoms	How have you been feeling in your mood? If I were to ask you to rate your mood on a scale from 1 to 10, what score would you give your mood now? Have others commented that you have been more irritable recently?	How has your energy level been? How has your sleep been? Are you still as energetic as ever despite the decreased amount of sleep? How has your appetite been?	Are you able to think clearly? Do you feel that there are many thoughts racing through your mind at any moment?	How long have you been feeling this way?
Eliciting hallucinations in all other modalities, eliciting thought disorders, eliciting passivity experiences	Auditory hallucinations Do you hear sounds or voices that others do not hear? How many voices could you hear? Are they as clear as our current conversation? What do they say?	Second-person auditory hallucinations Do they speak directly to you? Can you give me some examples of what they have been saying to you?	Third-person auditory hallucinations Do they refer to you as "he" or "she," much like a third person? Do they comment on your actions? Do they give you orders or commands as to what to do?	How do you feel when you hear them? Could there be any alternative explanation for these experiences that you have been having? Do you feel that your thoughts are being interfered with by an external force? Do you feel in control of your own actions and emotions?
Risk assessment— risk of excessive spending, intimacy, self-harm, violence	Have you engaged in any activities recently that might be dangerous? By that, I mean, have you been involved with the police recently?	Have you been spending more money than usual?	Have you been recently involved in any intimate relationships with others?	Have you been so troubled by all these that you have entertained thoughts of ending your life? Have you got into trouble with others around you?

Impact and coping mechanisms	How have you been coping with all these?	Have you made use of any substances, such as alcohol, to help you cope?	What about street drugs?	Have you been feeling this way since your antidepressants were recently adjusted?

Common pitfalls:

a. Failure to take control of the station.
b. Failure to elicit core hypomanic symptoms from the patient/failure to cover the range and depth of the station.
c. Failure to perform a complete risk assessment.
d. Failure to recognize the recent titration of antidepressants that may have precipitated the hypomania.

Information to candidates:

Name of patient: Mr Black

Mr Black, a 65-year-old man, has just been admitted to the orthopaedic ward after sustaining a fracture of his hip when he slipped and fell whilst bathing. He had his hip operation two days ago and is currently being nursed in the surgical high dependency unit. He has complained to the nurses that he has seen armed military officers around. He has often been aggressive and agitated, believing that the armed military officers around him might harm him.

Task: Please assess him for his psychopathology and perform a risk assessment.

Outline of station:

You are Mr Black, a 65-year-old man who has just been admitted to the orthopaedic ward. You have just recently undergone a hip replacement operation and are currently still in some pain. Things have not been the same for you as you have been seeing Spanish guerrillas whilst you are on the ward. You appeared to be very frightened and distressed by what you were seeing.

You start the station by telling the doctor this:

"There is no point for us to have a chat. Look, they are coming to get me. I think we better escape from this war zone right now."

You will then share (only if the doctor can take control of the interview and is empathetic) further information. You will share more about your visual and auditory hallucinations. You will then share some information about your alcohol history, stating that your last drink was around three days ago and that you have been a chronic drinker since your teenage years. Regarding risk, you will tell the doctor that you might think of absconding from the inpatient unit as this is too troubling for you. There might be a chance you might consider ending your life.

DOI: 10.1201/9781003313113-6

Approach: Be prepared that the patient may be difficult and reluctant to engage in an interview—take control by reassuring the patient and inviting him to sit down. If he refuses, sit down and start the station.

Starting off: "Hello, I am Dr Melvyn, one of the psychiatrists from the mental health unit. I received some information about you from my medical colleagues. Could you tell me more about what happened that led to your current admission?"

Alternatively, for a difficult patient:

"It seems to me that you are feeling very bothered now. Please let me reassure you that this is the hospital, and I'm one of the doctors. Could we have a chat?"

Eliciting core visual hallucinations	I can see that you seem to be quite distressed now. Are you able to tell me more about what you are seeing?	Do these people appear to be much smaller than usual? How long have you been troubled by these experiences? Have you had them before?	How do you feel when you see them? I understand that this must be a highly distressing situation for you. Do you feel that they are real? Is there any possibility of stopping them?	Why do you think they are troubling you? Do you have an explanation for these experiences? Could it be because you are not well now?
Elicit alcohol history if possible	I understand that you used alcohol before you came into the hospital. How often do you drink?	When did you first start to drink? Have you been increasing your alcohol intake recently?	Do you remember when you had your last drink? Was your last drink more than three days ago?	Have you tried to quit using alcohol previously? Were you successful?
Eliciting hallucinations in all other modalities, eliciting thought disorders, eliciting passivity experiences	**Auditory hallucinations** Do you hear sounds or voices that others do not hear? How many voices could you hear? Are they as clear as our current conversation? What do they say? Has there been anything wrong with your sense of smell recently?	**Second-person auditory hallucinations** Do they speak directly to you? Can you give me some examples of what they have been saying to you? Have you noticed that the food or drink seemed to have a different taste recently?	**Third-person auditory hallucinations** Do they refer to you as "he" or "she," much like a third person? Do they comment on your actions? Do they give you orders or commands as to what to do? Do you have any strange feelings in your body?	How do you feel when you hear them? Could there be any alternative explanation for these experiences that you have been having? Do you feel in control of your thoughts, emotions, and actions?

(Continued)

(Continued)

Check for orientation to time, place, person	Do you know where you are now?	Do you know roughly what time it is right now?	Do you know who I am?	
Risk assessment	With all these troubling experiences, have you thought of ending your life?	Have you thought of taking revenge on the people you think are troubling you?	Have you had any other symptoms? Were your hands trembling a lot? Do you recall if you have had a seizure/fit? Have you been feeling agitated in your mood?	

Common pitfalls:

a. Failure to take control of the station/failure to reassure the patient.
b. Failure to cover the range and depth of the station.
c. Failure to assess hallucinations in all other modalities.
d. Conducting the clinical interview standing throughout the entire seven minutes as the patient refuses to sit.

STATION 7
ANXIETY DISORDERS
(PANIC DISORDER WITH
AGORAPHOBIA)

Information to candidates:

Name of patient: Mrs Jones-Thomas

Mrs Jones-Thomas is a 35-year-old housewife. Her husband has brought her to the GP as she has had increasing anxiety about heading out of her house. Her GP has referred her over to the local mental health service for an assessment and potentially for psychological treatment.

Task: Please take a history to come to a diagnosis.

Outline of station:

You are Mrs Jones-Thomas, a 35-year-old housewife. You have been having increasing anxieties about leaving home, which started around six months ago. Six months ago, you were travelling on the tube when something nasty happened. The train broke down, and you were trapped in a tunnel with all the other passengers. There was not much ventilation, and you felt dizzy and nearly collapsed. That episode lasted for around 30 minutes before you were recused and managed to leave the tube. Ever since that episode, you have had increasing anxiety about leaving home. Even if you are with your husband, you worry that something similar might happen. Recently, you went out to shop for household items, and the same physical and psychological symptoms returned to trouble you. You recalled that during the last episode, you had palpitations, shortness of breath, giddiness, and fears of losing control and dying. Since then, you have been unable to get out of the house. You have resorted to purchasing items online, and you have also rejected all social invites by your friend. Your mood has been affected. You have not been using alcohol or any other substances to cope. You desperately want help. Begin the station by telling the doctor, "I think I have a serious problem. I don't think you could help me."

CASC Construct Table:

The CASC Construct Table is formatted such that candidates would be able adequately to cover both the range and depth of the assessment required in this station.

DOI: 10.1201/9781003313113-7

Approach: Be prepared that the patient may be difficult to engage at the start of the interview, as she has been feeling quite helpless about her situation. She might be quite anxious about coming to the doctor's appointment, and hence, if open questioning does not work, the candidate should consider closed-ended questions to elicit the core symptoms. **Starting off:** "Hello, I am Dr Melvyn, one of the psychiatrists from the mental health unit. I understand that you have been referred by your GP for anxiety symptoms. Could you tell me more?"				
History and eliciting core anxiety symptoms (physical and psychological)	Could you tell me how long this has been troubling you? Do you remember when this first started? Could you tell me more about your experiences during the first episode? Do you remember how long the episode lasted?	**Physical symptoms** Could you tell me more about your bodily symptoms during those episodes? — Palpitation — Sweating — Trembling — Dry mouth — Difficulty breathing — Chest pain — Nausea or stomach churning	**Psychological symptoms** When you have those bodily symptoms, what runs through your mind? Are you worried about losing control? Are you worried about dying or going crazy? Are you also afraid that something awful might happen?	How have you been in between those episodes? How frequently do these episodes occur now? Do you feel restless and keyed up, always on edge? Have you ever had exaggerated responses to minor surprises? Do you worry much about when the next attacks might occur? Are there specific situations in which these symptoms come on? For example, in situations which you cannot leave easily? Do you tend to avoid these situations?
Rule out other anxiety symptomatology and comorbidity	Do you worry a lot about everyday little things? Do you tend to get anxious when you must make conversations with people or give a presentation? Are there specific things that you are afraid of?	Do you have excessive checking or any washing behaviour? Do you have nightmare or flashbacks related to previous traumatic experiences?	I know this has been a difficult time for you. With all these going on, how has your mood been? Are you still able to keep up with your interests? What about your sleep and appetite?	

Impact and coping	How have these symptoms affected your life? Are you able to cope?	Have you used any alcohol to help you cope with your symptoms?	Have you used any other drugs to help you with all your symptoms?	Have you sought medical help previously?
Personal history	Is this the first time that you are seeing a psychiatrist? Does anyone in your family have any mental health problems?	How were things when you were a child? Were there any difficulties?	Could I know whether you have any chronic medical conditions? Have you had a history of thyroid problems? For the conditions that you have mentioned, are you on long-term medication?	How would you describe yourself in terms of your personality before all these symptoms started?

Common pitfalls:

a. Failure to engage the patient as she might be overtly anxious.
b. Failure to recognize the need to switch to closed-ended questioning if the patient does not answer open-ended questions.
c. Failure to cover the range and depth of the station/failure to rule out other anxiety conditions and assess mood.

Information to candidates:

Name of patient: Mr Lewis

Mr Lewis is a 30-year-old gentleman who has been referred to your clinic by his GP. He has recently visited his GP as he has been increasingly concerned about his upcoming marriage. He is reluctant to share further details with his GP. However, he has been insistent on getting medication to help him with his condition from the GP.

Task: Please take a history to come to a diagnosis. In addition, please elicit a history of possible aetiological factors.

Outline of station:

You are Mr Lewis, and your GP has referred you to see the psychiatrist. You are not very keen to see the psychiatrist as you do not want to be perceived as having any mental health problems, given that a major life event (your marriage) is coming up soon in two weeks. All you want from the GP is some medication that might calm you down during the event. Since you were young, you have been having difficulties in various social situations. You cannot give a presentation in front of others, and you dislike social gatherings and would avoid them at all costs. There are symptoms that come on during those social situations that have been particularly troubling for you previously. These include the sensation of blushing, dryness of mouth, palpitations, and the sensation of butterflies in your stomach. Because of your difficulties, since graduation, you have been forced to settle for a job as a chemist in the local lab. You always wanted to do finance and business management, but with your ongoing symptoms, you must give up that career option. You met your fiancée two years ago, and your relationship with her is good. She understands your problem, but she insists on having a church wedding (with approximately 200 guests), with which you have disagreed. All you want is a small event. What is more troubling for you is that you must give a speech during the wedding in front of others. You cannot perceive yourself doing that.

Your mood has been much affected by this. You still have retained interest and are still able to function at your workplace. You do not have any other anxiety symptoms, such as panic attacks or fear of going out. You do have a positive family history of mental health disorders, in which both your parents have anxiety disorders. You have not used any substances to cope with your current difficulties.

DOI: 10.1201/9781003313113-8

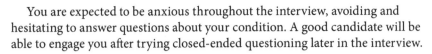

You are expected to be anxious throughout the interview, avoiding and hesitating to answer questions about your condition. A good candidate will be able to engage you after trying closed-ended questioning later in the interview.

CASC Construct Table:

The CASC Construct Table is formatted such that candidates would be able adequately to cover both the range and depth of the assessment required in this station.

Approach: Be prepared that the patient may be difficult to engage at the start of the interview as he has been feeling quite helpless about his situation. He might be pretty anxious about coming to the doctor's appointment; hence, if open questioning does not work, the candidate should consider closed-ended questioning to elicit the core symptoms. **Starting off:** "Hello, I am Dr Melvyn, one of the psychiatrists from the mental health unit. I understand that your GP has referred you for anxiety symptoms. Could you tell me more?"				
History and core anxiety symptoms	How long has this been troubling you for? Could I understand in what context or situations you feel this way?	Can you tell me more about your symptoms? What are the symptoms that you have in those situations? — Blushing — Dryness of mouth — Palpitations — Shaking — Urgency — Fear of micturition/ defecation	How do you respond when you feel this way?	
Psychosocial impact of anxiety symptoms	Do you tend to avoid certain situations?	Do you have any difficulties with your daily work?	Has this had any impact on your current relationships?	Is it true that, because of your current symptoms, you have resorted to avoiding certain situations, choosing to work in occupations that do not need much social interaction?
Rule out comorbidities	Do you worry a lot about everyday little things?	Do you have excessive checking or any washing behaviour?	I know this has been a difficult time for you.	Have you used any alcohol or any other drugs to help you cope with your current situation?

(Continued)

(Continued)

	Have you had panic attacks before? Do you have difficulties going out of the house? Are there specific things that you are afraid of?	Do you have nightmares or flashbacks related to previous traumatic experiences?	With all these going on, how has your mood been? Are you still able to keep up with your interests? What about your sleep and appetite?	
Personal history/ aetiology	Is this the first time that you are seeing a psychiatrist? Does anyone in your family have any mental health problems?	How were things when you were a child? Were there any difficulties?	Could I know whether you have any chronic medical conditions? Do you have a history of thyroid problems? For the conditions that you have mentioned, are you on long-term medication?	How would you describe yourself in terms of your personality before all these came on? Are you someone who always worries a lot?

Common pitfalls:

a. Failure to engage the patient as he might be overtly anxious.
b. Failure to recognize the need to switch to closed-ended questioning if the patient does not answer open-ended questions.
c. Failure to cover the range and depth of the station/failure to rule out other anxiety conditions and assess mood.
d. Failure to elicit the aetiological factors—the precipitating, the perpetuating, and the protective factors.

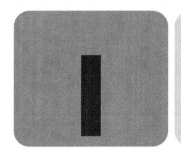

STATION 9
MENTAL STATE EXAMINATION (HOME LEAVE)

Information to candidates:

Name of patient: Mr Patel

Mr Patel is a 20-year-old gentleman who has been sectioned to the mental health unit after attempting to jump into the river three weeks ago. He shared with the team of doctors that he has been experiencing auditory hallucinations, command hallucinations, and delusional ideations for the past four months. The team doctors have diagnosed him with first episode of psychosis and have since started treatment for him. He is due to go on his home leave this weekend. The ward manager has requested for you to come and assess his mental state and his risk prior to him going on the planned home leave.

Task: Please perform a mental state examination and a relevant risk assessment.

Outline of station:

After attempting to jump into the River Thames, you were sectioned for admission to the mental health unit three weeks ago. You wanted to end your life at that time as you had been increasingly troubled by auditory hallucinations. You used to hear multiple voices that were making demeaning remarks and, at times, also commenting on your actions. The voices sounded as clear as any conversation you have had with others. The voices commanded you to jump into the river previously. You have also been increasingly troubled and have been feeling that there are spy cameras that are monitoring your actions. Your mood has been much affected by these experiences. You have been more settled whilst you are inpatient and since the commencement of medication.

You have been exercising quite a lot in the ward throughout your admission. Some residual voices are telling you to do so, as they tell you that the closer you get to the core of the Earth, the higher the chances of you becoming well again. You have plans to head out for your scheduled home leave with your sister as you are keen to find another river that is deeper than the previous one so that you could immerse yourself deep within and get rid of these experiences that have been troubling you. You do not think that this is dangerous.

CASC Construct Table:

The CASC Construct Table is formatted such that candidates would be able adequately to cover both the range and depth of the assessment required in this station.

DOI: 10.1201/9781003313113-9

Approach: Be prepared for a patient who might minimize his symptoms to go on home leave.

Starting off: "Hello, I am Dr Melvyn, one of the psychiatrists from the mental health unit. I understand that you are scheduled to go on your home leave. Could we have a chat as to how you have been?"

Home leave plans	I understand that you are due for a home leave today. Why do you wish to be allowed on home leave?	What plans do you have in mind? (Need to probe and get the patient to elaborate.)	When was the last time you went on home leave? How did you spend it? What happened when you were on home leave?	
Risk assessment— risk to self and others	Do you have plans to repeat what you did three weeks ago?	Have you felt that your life is no longer worth living? Do you have thoughts of ending your life? What plans do you have? (Assess history of suicide/self-harm.) Have you attempted suicide or hurt yourself before?	(If the patient vocalizes paranoid ideations.) Do you have any intentions to do anything nasty to the people who are troubling you? Do you have access to or do you plan to use any weapons?	Do you think you will return to the ward for continued treatment after your home leave?
Eliciting auditory hallucinations	**Auditory hallucinations** I understand the circumstances that led to your current admission. How have things changed? Do you still hear sounds or voices that others do not hear? How many voices could you hear? Are they as clear as our current conversation? What do they say?	**Second-person auditory hallucinations** Do they speak directly to you? Can you give me some examples of what they have been saying to you?	**Third-person auditory hallucinations** Do they refer to you as "he" or "she," much like a third person? Do they comment on your actions? Do they give you orders or commands as to what to do?	How do you feel when you hear them? Could there be any alternative explanation for these experiences that you have been having?
Eliciting delusions	I understand from the team that you have been exercising a lot in	How is it possible that exercising gives you more strength to deal	Are there any other alternative explanations for	Could it be that you have not yet been well?

	the ward. Could you tell me more about this?	with your experiences?	why you are thinking this way?	
Elicit thought disorders	**Thought interference** Do you feel that your thoughts are being interfered with? Who do you think is doing this?	**Thought insertion** Do you have thoughts in your head that you feel are not your own? Where do you think these thoughts come from?	**Thought broadcasting** Do you feel that your thoughts are being broadcasted such that others would know what you are thinking?	**Thought withdrawal** Do you feel that your thoughts are being taken away from your head by some external force?
Elicit passivity experiences	Do you feel in control of your own actions and emotions?	Do you feel that someone or something is trying to control you? Who or what do you think this would be?		
Impact of symptoms on mood and insight	I understand that this must be a difficult time for you. How have you been coping?	Since admission till now, how has your mood been? Are you still interested in things you used to enjoy?	I understand that the team doctors have started you on some medication. Did they share with you what might be wrong with you? Do you believe them?	Do you know why you need the medication?

Common pitfalls:

a. Failure to engage with a patient who might be minimizing his symptoms.
b. Failure to cover the range and depth of the station.
c. Failure to perform an adequate risk assessment—need to take into consideration risk of harm to self and others and risk of absconding and not returning to the ward.
d. Failure to assess the history of suicide/self-harm episodes and their severity/lethality.

STATION 10
DEPRESSION WITH
PSYCHOTIC FEATURES

Information to candidates:

Name of patient: Ms Johnson

You are the core trainee-3 on call. Your medical colleagues from the emergency services have asked you to help assess a 70-year-old female who has just been transferred to their service via ambulance. You have been informed that she has tried to burn herself alive in her backyard, but her neighbours noticed it and called the police. You have been told that she has been vocalizing to the medical doctors that she thinks she is already dead and does not want them to do anything for her. Your medical colleagues have done the necessary blood investigations and have deemed her to be medically stable.

Task: Please ask the patient to learn more about her abnormal beliefs and perform an appropriate risk assessment.

Outline of station:

You are Ms Johnson, and you regret that your attempt to burn yourself in your backyard has not been successful. You feel that your neighbours are troublemakers and that they should not have contacted the police and the ambulance. You are convinced that you are already dead, and your plan today was to get rid of your physical body as you know that it is rotting away already. You are convinced that, around one month ago, when you awoke, you saw the angel at the foot of your bed, which was a clear sign for you that you were dead. You will begin the station telling the candidate "I am dead" and "You are talking to my soul" and repeat it no matter what the candidate asks or says. If the candidate asks, "What happened before you realized you're dead?" and appears to be empathetic, you will be willing to engage more. You will have absolutely no eye contact with the candidate, and your mood is very low.

You will share with the candidate that you have been feeling low in your spirits since a few months ago, when you were made redundant at your workplace and when your youngest son passed on from a silent heart attack. Since then, your mood has been pervasively low, and you have no interest in activities that you used to find enjoyable. Your sleep and appetite are affected. You have active ideations of doing something similar again on discharge as you cannot envision living on.

CASC Construct Table:

The CASC Construct Table is formatted such that candidates would be able adequately to cover both the range and depth of the assessment required in this station.

DOI: 10.1201/9781003313113-10

Approach: Be prepared for a patient who is very depressed and delusional and not willing to engage. Demonstrate empathy, and if the patient keeps insisting that she is dead, please ask her "What happened before you died?" to attempt to elicit the range and depth of information required in the station.

Starting off: "Hello, I am Dr Melvyn, one of the psychiatrists from the mental health unit. Could you tell me more about what has happened?"

Eliciting nihilistic delusions and challenging delusions	It does sound like things have been difficult for you. How long have you been feeling this way for?	What does it mean when you say you are dead? Do you feel that parts of your body are rotting? Was that the reason that led you to do what you did today? How convinced are you that you are dead?	How did you know that you are dead? Did anything happen that led you to believe so?	How is it possible for us to be having a conversation now if you are already dead? Could there be an alternative explanation to all these?
Eliciting depressive symptoms	Key question: Could you tell me more about how things have been for you before you died?	With all these going on, how was your mood? Are you able to enjoy things you used to enjoy?	How has your sleep been? Have there been any problems with your appetite? What were your energy levels like?	Have you had thoughts that life was not worth living? What are your plans for the future?
Eliciting psychotic symptoms?	Have there been times when you are alone by yourself and you have been bothered by unusual experiences? Do you hear voices when no one is around?	Do you feel that your thoughts are being interfered with?	Do you feel in control of your own emotions?	Do you feel in control of your actions?
Risk assessment	This must be an extremely difficult time for you.	What were your intentions when you tried to burn yourself today?	"Do you still have thoughts of ending your life right now? What plans do you have in mind?	Is there anything that will prevent you from doing so?

Common pitfalls:

a. Failure to engage with a patient who is supposed to be extremely depressed in this station.

b. Failure to cover the range and depth of the station (failure to elicit both the depressive and the psychotic symptoms and adequately challenge the delusional beliefs).

c. Failure to perform an adequate risk assessment—includes harm to self, others, and damage to property.

STATION 11
DEPRESSION WITH
PSYCHOTIC FEATURES

Information to candidates:

Name of patient: Mrs Beale

You are the core trainee-3 on call. You have been asked to assess a 55-year-old female who has been brought into the emergency services by the police. You received information that she has attempted to surrender herself today to the police as she is convinced that she committed a terrible crime many years ago. The medics have performed the basic bloodwork for her and have cleared her medically.

Task: Please ask the patient to find out more about the abnormal beliefs she has and perform an appropriate risk assessment.

Outline of station:

You are Mrs Beale, a 55-year-old female. You have decided to surrender yourself to the police station today as you strongly believe that you committed a serious crime and mistake years ago. This came to your realization a month ago when you were watching a television documentary about the adoption of children. This reminded you that you have intentionally left out the name of your daughter's father on her birth certificate as you had a conflict with your husband back then and decided not to include his name. You know that your daughter's marriage is undergoing a tough time, and you believe that this is all because you intentionally left out the name of your husband. You have told your husband about your concerns, but he does not believe you.

Your mood has been low for the past month or so. You cannot enjoy the things you used to enjoy. The house is in a state of a mess as you have barely sufficient energy to do the housework. Your sleep is disrupted, and your appetite is poor as you constantly ruminate over the serious crime that you have committed. Recently, you have not dared to watch the television as you feel that the people on the television programmes might talk about your crime. At times, when you are alone, you hear voices, which sound like those of your husband, asking you to surrender yourself to the police for the serious mistake you have committed. You feel your life is meaningless and have had passive ideations of suicide. You are very afraid that you might do something to end your life as this is troubling you very much.

CASC Construct Table:

The CASC Construct Table is formatted such that candidates would be able adequately to cover both the range and depth of the assessment required in this station.

DOI: 10.1201/9781003313113-11

Approach: Be prepared for a patient who might be quite restless, anxious, and preoccupied with thoughts that she has indeed committed a major crime. Use empathetic statements to engage the patient.

Starting off: "Hello, I am Dr Melvyn, one of the psychiatrists from the mental health unit. Could you tell me more about what happened prior to your current admission?"

Eliciting delusional beliefs and challenging the belief	I could see that you looked very distressed. Could you tell me more about what has been troubling you?	Could you tell me more as to why you are feeling this way? Did anything remind you of what happened previously?	Do you feel that you are guilty and responsible for all that has happened to your daughter's relationship? Could there be any other alternative explanations for this?	Could it be possible that your daughter already has some marital issues to begin with?
Eliciting depressive symptoms	With all these ongoing, how was your mood? Are you able to enjoy things you used to enjoy?	How has your sleep been? Have there been any problems with your appetite? How were your energy levels like?	Have you had thoughts that life was not worth living? What are your plans for the future?	
Eliciting psychotic symptoms?	Have there been times when you are alone and you have been bothered by unusual experiences?	Do you feel that your thoughts are being interfered with?	Do you feel in control of your own emotions?	Do you feel in control of your own actions?
Risk assessment	This must be an extremely difficult time for you.	Have you had thoughts of ending your life previously?	Do you still have thoughts of ending your life right now?	What plans do you have in mind? Is there anything that will prevent you from doing so?

Common pitfalls:

a. Failure to engage with the patient.
b. Failure to challenge her delusional beliefs adequately.
c. Failure to cover the range and depth of the station (failure to elicit both the depressive and the psychotic symptoms).
d. Failure to perform an adequate risk assessment.

STATION 12
DELUSION OF LOVE/
EROTOMANIA

Information to candidates:

Name of patient: Mr Jordan

You are the core trainee-3 on call, and you have been informed by the emergency services receptionist to evaluate a gentleman who has turned up unexpectedly and now demanding to see the nurse who treated him one week ago.

Task: Please speak to the patient and assess his psychopathology. In addition, please perform an assessment of risk.

Outline of station:

You are Mr Jordan, and you have returned to the emergency department today, requesting to see the nurse (whom you call "Sarah") who attended to you around one week ago. You are insistent on seeing her today as you believe that she is in love with you. You are extremely convinced about this, from the special way that she treated you three weeks ago and from the way she smiled at you. You are keen to meet up with her today and take this relationship further. In addition, you have made some plans of what you wish to do if she is willing to go on a date with you. You want to have a good meal with her and then take it further from that. You desire intimacy and have been thinking of chaining her to the bed and having intimacy with her. You have done this before with your previous two other girlfriends, who have since left you. There was one occasion in which one of your girlfriends reported you to the police for the acts that you had done against her.

You do not know much about the nurse whom you met three weeks ago. All you know is that she works in the hospital and that her shift is usually around this time. You do not have additional details such as where she stays or her telephone number. You have not attempted to stalk or follow her home.

You are very insistent on meeting the nurse today. You are upset that the receptionist could not facilitate this. Now, you think that it is absurd that you must meet up with a psychiatrist to discuss this with him/her. You have been holding onto a bag, which contains a knife within, and you would consider using the knife to deal with anyone who interferes with your plan.

CASC Construct Table:

The CASC Construct Table is formatted such that candidates would be able adequately to cover both the range and depth of the assessment required in this station.

DOI: 10.1201/9781003313113-12

Approach: The patient is expected to be very demanding and insist on meeting up with the nurse. He might be aggressive and hostile as well. Pay attention to non-verbal cues as he might be holding a bag with a knife within. Make use of the initial few minutes to establish rapport.

Starting off: "Hello, I am Dr Melvyn, one of the psychiatrists from the mental health unit. I understand that you have come here today requesting to see one of my psychiatric nurses. Could you tell me more?"

Introduction and establishment of rapport	I understand that you are very keen to see Sarah. However, it has been a surprise that you have come unexpectedly today.	I am here to help you, but firstly, I need to understand a bit more. Could you tell me more?	How did you know Sarah?	Could you tell me more about when you first met her?	
Explore and challenge existing delusions	What is your relationship with Sarah? When did you first feel that Sarah started to love you?	What made you think so? How do you know that she is indeed in love with you?	Has she told you anything? How likely is this feeling?	From my understanding, you only met her once. Could this be possible?	Could it not be possible that this is how she is, and she treats all patients in the same way?
Knowledge about victim	Thanks for sharing with me so patiently. Could you tell me how much you know about Sarah?	Apart from knowing that she works here, do you know where she stays?	Do you know her mobile number? Have you looked her up in the local phone directory?	Have you ever followed her home before?	Do you know whether she is in a current relationship?
Explore and assess other psychiatric pathology	How has your mood been thus far? Do you still have an interest in what you love to do? What do you do for work, and whom do you live with?	Have there been any changes in your sleep or your appetite recently?	Do you feel more self-confident as compared to others? Do you feel that you have some special abilities that others do not have?	Have you ever had strange experiences, such as hearing voices when no one is there or seeing things when no one is there?	Have you used substances like alcohol or other street drugs to help you cope with your anxiety previously?
Forensic history and risk assessment	Could you tell me more about what plans you have in mind if you are able to meet Sarah tonight?	Is this the first relationship you have had?	Why were the police involved?	What will happen if Sarah decides not to meet you?	It has been quite a surprise for us that you turned up today. What if

	Do you have plans to get intimate with her?	You mentioned your previous girlfriends. Could you tell me more about how those relationships went?	Have you been involved with the police for other reasons?	Would you have thoughts of ending it all?	we say that we need more information from Sarah before we allow her to see you?

Common pitfalls:

a. Failure to engage with a difficult patient.
b. Failure to challenge his delusional beliefs adequately.
c. Failure to cover the range and depth of the station (failure to elicit more background information from the patient regarding his knowledge about the nurse, failure to elicit and consider other psychiatric diagnoses).
d. Failure to ask questions about his previous forensic history.
e. Failure to ask about drugs and substance usage.
f. Failure to perform an adequate risk assessment.

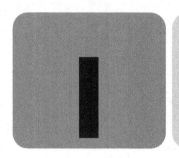

Information to candidates:

Name of patient: Mr Nair

> You are a core trainee-3, and the mentioned patient has come to see you as he has some concerns. From the previous medical records, you know that he has had a previous diagnosis of ADHD. He is worried about his participation in an upcoming World Cup as he has been having difficulties focusing on his training.

Task: Please speak to the patient and elicit a history to support his previous diagnosis of ADHD. In addition, please also identify his current problems and address any concerns that he might have. Please do not perform a mental state examination.

Outline of station:

> You are Mr Nair, and you have come to see the doctor as you are very concerned about whether you will be able to participate in an upcoming World Cup. You have been having difficulties focusing on the training. You were previously diagnosed with ADHD in childhood. Your parents had told you that when you were six years old, you had symptoms of inattention, hyperactivity, and impulsiveness. You frequently got into trouble in school. A child psychiatrist assessed you and started you on medication. You stopped the medication after two years as there were some abnormalities on your liver function tests. You're concerned about your current symptoms. You're worried about being on stimulant medication as you are concerned about how it will affect your eligibility. You have not used any other drugs to help you cope with your symptoms. You expect the doctor to be empathetic and listen to your concerns.

CASC Construct Table:

The CASC Construct Table is formatted such that candidates would be able adequately to cover both the range and depth of the assessment required in this station.

DOI: 10.1201/9781003313113-13

Approach: The patient is likely to be very anxious about his eligibility to participate in the upcoming international competition. Demonstrate empathy and establish rapport with the patient, reassuring him that you need more information prior to commenting on whether he is eligible.

Starting off: "Hello, I am Dr Melvyn, one of the psychiatrists from the mental health unit. I understand that you came to see us today as you have some concerns. Could you tell me more?"

Identification of current problem (core ADHD symptoms currently)	(Inattentive symptoms are common in adult ADHD) Can you tell me more about the symptoms that you have currently?	Do you find yourself being inattentive at times? Could you give me some examples of this? Are you also easily distractable?	Are you able to cope with the tasks you are assigned or plan to do? Do you tend to lose things easily?
Identification of the current core symptoms on his level of functioning	I understand that it has not been easy for you. How have your current symptoms affected you in terms of your functioning?	Are you able to function at your current workplace? Have there been any specific problems to date? Have you needed to change jobs? Did you find yourself better able to cope if you were to work shorter hours?	How have things been at home? Have your current symptoms had any impact on your existing relationships?
Identification of childhood history to support a previous diagnosis of ADHD	Can you tell me more about when your ADHD was first diagnosed? Do you remember what the main problems were back then?	Hyperactivity symptoms: Do you find yourself always restless and always on the go? Was it difficult to queue and wait for your turn? Impulsiveness symptoms: Are there times to when you did things on the spur of the moment? Have there been times in which you answer before others finished their questions?	Did you have any other difficulties when you were younger besides ADHD? Has your academic performance been affected as well? Could you tell me more about the previous treatments that you have had? Do you remember the reasons why the medication that was previously started for you was stopped?
Consideration of other psychiatric comorbidities	How has your mood been recently? Are you still able to have an interest in things that you used to be interested in?	Have you used any substances such as alcohol or drugs to help you cope with your current condition?	

(Continued)

(Continued)

Risk assessment	Have you been involved with the police previously? Could you tell me more?	Have you or people around you noticed that you have been more irritable recently? Have you got into any trouble with others?	Do you find yourself being more impulsive and more reckless when driving?
Address current concerns	I understand that you are concerned about how you could cope with the new demands at work. I can help you with a medical memo, but before that I may need to contact your previous psychiatrist and any other doctors to get more information. Will that be all right?	I understand that you would like to be considered for medication that might help your inattentiveness. Have you heard of any ADHD medication? Medication for ADHD do not cure the underlying condition but help with symptoms management. There are two types of medications commonly used: stimulants and non-stimulants.	Stimulant medication (such as methylphenidate) works by increasing the levels of dopamine, which, for individuals with ADHD, helps improve concentration and reduce hyperactivity. There are both short and long-acting stimulants. Stimulants are not suitable for individuals with heart conditions and high blood pressure. They need to be carefully considered if one has any pre-existing psychiatric conditions or history of drug abuse. Some of the common side effects one might experience include that of poor appetite, weight loss, insomnia, tics, and elevated blood pressure. Non-stimulants (Atomoxetine) work by increasing the levels of noradrenaline in the brain, thus helping with ADHD symptoms. They should be considered one experience side effects or have contraindications to the use of stimulants. Some of the common side effects include lethargy, headache, dizziness, nausea and vomiting, and mood swings.

Common pitfalls:

a. Failure to engage with a patient who might be very anxious initially and keeps requesting help with a medical memo.
b. Failure to elicit current core ADHD symptoms.
c. Failure to assess the impact of current core ADHD symptoms on his level of functioning.
d. Failure to elicit comprehensive childhood history of ADHD.
e. Being unsure of the clinical guidelines and recommendations for the treatment of adult ADHD.
f. Failure to recognize that stimulants may be detected on a urine drug screen and failure to present alternatives to stimulants.

Information to candidates:

Name of patient: Mr Chan

You are a core trainee-3, and you are running the outpatient specialist service. You have received a referral from your cardiology colleague, who has referred a 23-year-old gentleman to you. The referral letter states that the gentleman has frequent chest pain with palpitations and the cardiologist has done a whole host of investigations, all of which were normal. The gentleman, Mr Chan, remains very concerned about his condition nevertheless and feels that the cardiologist might be missing something.

Task: Please speak to the patient and elicit a detailed history from him to arrive at a diagnosis. Please also elicit the relevant aetiological factors. Finally, please address his concerns and expectations and discuss the treatment options.

Outline of station:

You are Mr Chan, a 23-year-old university student. Over the past 3 months or so, you have been troubled by frequent sudden onset of the following symptoms: chest pain, palpitations, and shortness of breath. These physical symptoms are associated with worries that you might lose control of yourself and even faint during the episode. These episodes usually come on suddenly, and the peak of the symptoms usually lasts for around 15 minutes or so. You worry very much about when the next attack might come on. You do not have any past medical history of note, but you have since consulted several doctors, and none of them could give you a definitive answer as to why you have these symptoms.

You worry that this might be a heart condition which the cardiologist has missed. You have an uncle who passed on at the age of 30 due to sudden cardiac arrest. Since you were young, your family has been very health conscious. In addition, you are someone who worries a lot in terms of your personality. You get the attacks whether you are at home or in crowded spaces. You appeared to be anxious about your current health condition, but you are not depressed. You do not have any specific fears or fears of presenting in front of others. You do not have obsessional thoughts or compulsive acts. You seek to understand from the psychiatrist more about the treatment of the current condition—both medical treatment and talking therapy.

DOI: 10.1201/9781003313113-14

CASC Construct Table:

The CASC Construct Table is formatted such that candidates would be able adequately to cover both the range and depth of the assessment required in this station.

Approach: Be prepared that the patient may be difficult to engage at the start of the interview as he might not want to be seen by a psychiatrist. Be empathetic towards the patient, stating that you are involved in his care as part of a collaborative approach to help him with his symptoms. Starting off: "Hello, I am Dr Melvyn, one of the psychiatrists from the mental health unit. I understand that the cardiologist has referred you. Could you tell me more?"				
History and eliciting core anxiety symptoms (physical and psychological)	Could you tell me how long this has been troubling you? Do you remember when this first started? Could you tell me more about your experiences during the first episode? Do you remember how long the episode lasted?	**Physical symptoms** Could you tell me more about your bodily symptoms during those episodes? — Palpitation — Sweating — Trembling — Dry mouth — Difficulty breathing — Chest pain — Nausea or stomach churning	**Psychological symptoms** When you have those bodily symptoms, what runs through your mind? Are you worried about losing control? Are you worried about dying or going crazy? Are you also afraid that something awful might happen?	How have you been in between those episodes? How frequently do these episodes occur now? Do you feel restless and keyed up, always on edge? Have you ever had exaggerated responses to minor surprises? Do you worry much about when the next attack might occur? Are there specific situations to which these symptoms come on? For example, in situations which you cannot leave easily? Do you tend to avoid these situations?
Rule out medical comorbidity and other anxiety symptomatology	I understand that the cardiologist has done a series of tests for you. Are you aware of the test results? I know that you are very concerned about your current	Apart from what you have shared, do you worry a lot about everyday little things? Do you tend to get anxious when you must make	Do you have excessive checking or any washing behaviour? Do you have nightmares or flashbacks	I know this has been a difficult time for you. With all these going on, how has your mood been? Are you still able to keep up with your interests?

(Continued)

(Continued)

	symptoms. Could I find out a bit more so that I could help you?	conversations with people or give a presentation? Are there specific things that you are afraid of?	related to previous traumatic experiences?	What about your sleep and appetite?
Impact and coping	How have these symptoms affected your life? Are you able to cope?	Have you used any alcohol to help you cope with your symptoms?	Have you used any other drugs to help you with all your symptoms?	Have you sought medical help previously?
Personal history	Is this the first time that you are seeing a psychiatrist? Does anyone in your family have any mental health problems? Have there been any recent changes in the family? Have there been any recent significant life events?	How were things when you were a child? Were there any difficulties?	Could I know whether you have any chronic medical conditions? For the conditions that you have mentioned, are you on long-term medication? Does anyone in the family have any past medical history?	How would you describe yourself in terms of your personality before all these came on?
Diagnosis	Thanks for sharing with me your concerns.	From the symptoms that you have shared, it seems to me that you have an anxiety disorder called panic attack. Have you heard about it before? How much do you know about panic disorder?	Thank you for sharing your understanding with me. Perhaps, I can take some of your time to explain in more detail what a panic disorder is all about.	Mention fight and flight action and how stimulation of the autonomic system causes the sympathetic overdrive.
Clarification of possible aetiology factors	You seemed to be concerned about what precipitated this entire episode.	From my assessment, some of the possible factors include the following:		

		a. Recent stressors b. Presence of a family history of psychiatric disorder c. Premorbid anxious personality		
Treatment options	Panic disorder is a relatively common disorder. There are various treatment options, both medication and talking therapies. Which one do you want me to speak about first?	There are medicines that could help. Benzodiazepines/ hypnotics and beta-blockers like propranolol are generally helpful for acute attacks and short-term use. Propranolol helps reduce palpitations (if one does not have any underlying asthma). Antidepressants like SSRIs could also help one cope with panic attacks	In addition to medication, it might be helpful to consider talking therapy. The commonest talking therapy is that CBT. Have you heard of that before?	Perhaps, let me share a bit more about CBT. In CBT, cognitive therapy helps in modifying thoughts on anticipatory anxiety; behavioural therapy focuses on deep breathing and relaxation exercises to help one deal with the symptoms.

Common pitfalls:
  a. Failure to engage a patient who might be reluctant to speak to a psychiatrist as he thinks that his symptoms are medical in nature.
  b. Failure to elicit a full history of the presenting complaint—not eliciting information such as the duration of the symptoms, the onset, etc.
  c. Failure to cover the aetiological factors that might contribute to his current illness.
  d. Inadequate usage and demonstration of empathy to reassure the patient throughout the interview.
  e. Discussing only the pharmacological management option and not the psychological treatment option.
  f. The patient may ask how being anxious psychologically causes the physical symptoms—it is important to be able to explain the phenomenon adequately.

Information to candidates:

Name of patient: Ms Woods

You are a core trainee-3, and you are running the outpatient service. You are seeing a 30-year-old female, Ms Woods, who has a chronic history of schizophrenia, which was first diagnosed at the age of 20. She has been on long-term psychotropic medication, with which she has been compliant. She is currently on risperidone 5 mg. She came today as she has been increasingly concerned that she has not been having her menses for the last year, and you have organized some blood tests before the appointment today. The blood tests revealed that her prolactin levels are currently 880 mIU/L.

Task: Please explain to Ms Woods the blood test results. Please consider taking a history if necessary to check for prolactin-related symptoms. Please address all her concerns about the future management of her condition. Please do not perform a mental state examination.

Outline of station:

You are Ms Woods, and you have been diagnosed with schizophrenia since the age of 20. You have been sectioned for inpatient admission on three occasions, and your last relapse was around three years ago. You have managed well thus far as you have been compliant with your psychotropic medication—risperidone 5 mg. However, over the past year, you have noticed that you have not had your menses. This is your main concern. In addition to not having your menses, you do have other troubling symptoms, to which you will disclose only if the doctor is sensitive and demonstrate empathy. You do have a milky discharge from your breast occasionally. You want to know the results of your blood test that the doctor has mentioned he will organize for you, and you want to know whether the symptoms that you are having are related to the medication. You also wish to know the long-term side effects of the medication. You wish to discuss with the doctor how best to manage your condition—would a switch of medication be ideal, and what is the risk?

CASC Construct Table:

The CASC Construct Table is formatted such that candidates would be able adequately to cover both the range and depth of the assessment required in this station.

DOI: 10.1201/9781003313113-15

Approach: Be prepared that the patient might be very anxious about her blood test results. She might be shocked to know that her blood test results are abnormal. It is important to reassure her and to demonstrate adequate empathy and sensitivity when asking her about other prolactin-related clinical symptoms.

Starting off: "Hello, I am Dr Melvyn, one of the psychiatrists from the mental health unit. I understand that you are here today to find out more about the blood test which was done?"

Clarification of blood test results and explanation of likely causes for deranged results	Did you come with anyone today? I like to share with you that one of the results of your blood test is abnormal (the prolactin levels). Would it be all right if I go on?	Based on the results obtained, it does show that your prolactin levels are outside of the normal range. This means that you have a higher-than-normal amount of this hormone called prolactin. Have you heard about prolactin before? Prolactin is a hormone which is produced by your pituitary gland. It is responsible for breast development and milk production after childbirth. Prolactin also regulates the menstrual cycle.	I understand that you are very concerned about the results. In hyperprolactinemia, there is too much prolactin produced. This might affect the production of other hormones, such as oestrogen and progesterone, and might result in ovulation changes or irregular and missed periods. Can I clarify that you are only on risperidone 5 mg for your schizophrenia? Very often, the high prolactin levels might be due to the antipsychotic medication that you are on. Other common causes include these: a. Hypothyroidism b. Stress c. Local irritation of the chest wall d. Pituitary tumours
Eliciting clinical features of hyperprolactinemia	I understand that your menstrual cycle has been abnormal for the past year. Have there been any other bodily changes?	I'd need to ask you some sensitive personal questions to help you with your condition. Apart from the menstrual changes, have there been occasions where you have discharge from your breasts?	Have there been any times to when you have had other bodily symptoms, such as headaches, blurred vision, weakness, and numbness of your limbs?

(Continued)

(Continued)

		Have you noticed any changes in your intimacy recently?	If you do experience other symptoms, we could refer you to a medical specialist for more investigative checks, which might include a magnetic resonance scan of your brain to exclude the possibility of a tumour.
Clarification of long-term side effects	It does seem like the bodily changes you are experiencing are due to the high levels of prolactin caused by the medication you have been on.	Over the long term, there might be a risk of osteoporosis—by that I mean your bones get weaker.	I'm sorry, but there might also be a possible increase in the risk of breast cancer.
Discussion of the management plan	There are several options available to help you with these difficulties.	We could consider a switch to another non-prolactin elevating drug, such as antipsychotics like olanzapine and aripiprazole. Have you heard of them before?	The other option would be to add newer antipsychotics like aripiprazole to your existing treatment regimen. Other medicines that could be considered are cabergoline and bromocriptine.

Common pitfalls:

   a. Failure to explain the results simplistically to the patient whilst being reassuring to the patient.

   b. Failure to explain hyperprolactinemia in a simplistic manner.

   c. Failure to elicit core symptoms and to rule out possible neurological causes.

   d. Failure to clarify the long-term side effects of having a raised prolactin level.

   e. Failure to offer plausible treatment alternatives, which includes changing the antipsychotics or commencement of other medication to reduce the levels.

STATION 16
EXPLAIN CLOZAPINE TREATMENT

Information to candidates:

Name of patient: Mr Khan

Mr Khan has been diagnosed with schizophrenia since the age of 20 years. He has been compliant with his medication, but he still has had numerous involuntary admissions for relapse of his underlying condition. He has tried several antipsychotics from the typical and the atypical classes. Further collaborative history obtained from the family revealed that his medication is supervised, and he has not had any recent substance or drug usage. His case has been discussed with the other members of the multidisciplinary team. The ward consultant has decided to start treating him with clozapine as he seemed to have treatment-resistant schizophrenia. The ward consultant hopes that you could discuss more about clozapine with him as it is likely to be beneficial for his condition.

Task: Please explain to Mr Khan the rationale for the team's decision to start him on an alternative antipsychotic known as clozapine. Please explore his concerns as well as his expectations.

Outline of station:

You are Mr Khan, and you have been diagnosed with schizophrenia since you were 20 years old. You have had three previous admissions to the inpatient unit for stabilization following a relapse of your condition. You do not use any illegal substances and have been compliant with the recommended medication dosages. You feel helpless as the doctors have tried several antipsychotics, but they have not been beneficial for your condition. You are keen to hear about this new medication that the core trainee will be discussing with you. You have only a limited understanding of this medication as you do know of friends who have been on it. You have your concerns—you wish to know more about the medication, how the medication could help you, the side effects of the medication, and the necessary monitoring process that needs to be done when you are on the medication. You are concerned about the side effects of the medication. In addition, you are very concerned about the risk associated with relapse if you happen to have missed doses of the medication. You wish to ask the doctor whether you could take alcohol with the medication too.

CASC Construct Table:

The CASC Construct Table is formatted such that candidates would be able adequately to cover both the range and depth of the assessment required in this station.

DOI: 10.1201/9781003313113-16

Approach: Be prepared that the patient might be extremely anxious about the commencement of this new medication called clozapine. He might be feeling helpless, given that he has tried quite a few typical and atypical antipsychotics previously. Try to engage the patient and start off by asking his understanding of the new medication.

Starting off: "Hello, I am Dr Melvyn, one of the psychiatrists from the mental health unit. The team wants me to discuss with you the option of starting a new medication called clozapine. Will that be all right?

Clarify the rationale for the commencement of clozapine	Could you tell me more about your understanding of clozapine?	Perhaps let me share more about clozapine. Clozapine is an antipsychotic medication that is commonly used to treat patients with treatment-resistant schizophrenia. Schizophrenia is deemed treatment-resistant when three or more medicines have been tried and have not helped with the condition.	In schizophrenia, neurochemicals like dopamine are overactive and in excess. Clozapine helps to block some of the dopamine in the brain, and hence it will help you with your symptoms. Studies have shown that approximately every 6 out of 10 people do benefit from the commencement of clozapine, and we are hopeful it will help you as well.
Describe the investigations necessary for the initiation of clozapine and the rationale	I understand that you're concerned as to when you could start clozapine. Prior to starting clozapine, we need to do some blood tests for you, as well as register you with the Clozapine Patient Monitoring Service.	As clozapine could cause a reduction in the white blood cells (which are the cells necessary to fight off any infections) in around two to three in every hundred people taking it, it is a necessity for us to do a baseline blood count. We will need you to repeat the blood tests every week for the first 18 weeks. If things go well, we will then do the blood tests every two weeks for the remainder of the year.	Apart from the baseline blood count (full blood count), we will do other blood tests and a baseline heart tracing of your heart rhythm before commencing you on clozapine.
Explain common side effects and highlight dangerous side effects	As with all other medication, clozapine has side effects. Some of the more common side effects include	Our team will start your clozapine at the lowest dose and increase the medication gradually to	Apart from the side effects previously mentioned, some of the rarer side effects

	those of sedation, lowering of blood pressure and increased salivation. Some patients also complain of weight gain and constipation.	minimize these side effects.	include a reduction in the total number of white blood cells in the body, which will affect your body's ability to fight off an infection. Also, there is an increased chance of fits/seizures for patients who are on high dose of clozapine. We need your help to seek medical advice immediately if you are feeling unwell or down with an infection.
Clarify other concerns	Clozapine is an antipsychotic medication and is not addictive in nature. You do not have to take more of the same dose to get the same effect over time.	The treatment duration varies for every individual. We will monitor your symptoms and advise you accordingly.	We do not advise you to stop the medication, for your symptoms might return. We understand your concerns about missing a dose. Please take the medication as prescribed if you have missed a dose within 24 hours. Do not double the dose. Please let us know if you miss the dose for more than 24 hours. It would not be advisable for you to mix alcohol and clozapine as it might cause increased drowsiness.

Common pitfalls:

a. Failure to allay the anxiety of the patient regarding his concerns about the new medication and engage him in the interview.
b. Failure to explain a simplified concept of "treatment-resistant schizophrenia."
c. Failure to convince the patient to try out clozapine, as there is too much emphasis on the side effect profile. Remember to mention how effective clozapine has been for patients with treatment-resistant schizophrenia.
d. Failure to mention the need for regular blood checking and dose titration for clozapine.
e. Failure to address all the concerns of the patient. (Please leave some time at the end of the interview to ask the patient whether he has further questions.)

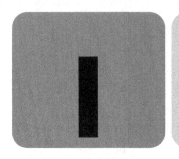

Information to candidates:

Name of patient: Ms Banerjee

Ms Banerjee is a 35-year-old female who has been suffering from depressive disorder since the age of 22. She has tried several antidepressants, but they have not been helpful for her. She still suffers from frequent relapses that require inpatient stabilization because of the risk of self-harm. She is currently on citalopram. The team has discussed her condition, and the team consultant wants to consider augmenting her existing antidepressant with lithium. You are the core trainee-3 in the team, and your team consultant wants you to discuss this with her.

Task: Please explain to Ms Banerjee the rationale for the augmentation of her existing antidepressant and address all her concerns.

Outline of station:

You are Ms Banerjee, and this is your third admission to the inpatient unit this year. You have been diagnosed with a depressive disorder since the age of 22. You have tried several types of medications, but none of the antidepressants seemed to help you much with your condition. You still have frequent relapses, which require you to be admitted, as whenever you have a relapse, you will be suicidal. You have been on citalopram 20 mg for the past six months, and you have not improved much on this new medication. Your mood is persistently low, and you are always feeling tired. You cannot keep up with any of your interests at all. You understand that the team's doctor is here to discuss with you more about using another medication to enhance your current antidepressant. You're keen to find out more.

Regarding the new medication, you are especially concerned about the side effects of the medication. If you hear that it might cause kidney toxicity, you express deep concern as your father passed on due to kidney failure. You wish to know when you could start the medication, the monitoring process prior to starting, and what you need to do if you are taking the medication. You have concerns pertaining to whether the medication is addictive and whether you could use alcohol whilst on the medication. You wonder whether the medication might affect the chance of you getting pregnant.

CASC Construct Table:

The CASC Construct Table is formatted such that candidates would be able adequately to cover both the range and depth of the assessment required in this station.

DOI: 10.1201/9781003313113-17

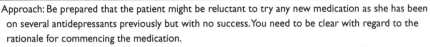

Approach: Be prepared that the patient might be reluctant to try any new medication as she has been on several antidepressants previously but with no success. You need to be clear with regard to the rationale for commencing the medication.

Starting off: "Hello, I am Dr Melvyn, one of the psychiatrists from the mental health unit. The team wants me to discuss with you the option of starting a new medication called lithium. Will that be all right?"

Clarify the rationale for the commencement of lithium	Have you heard about lithium before? What is your understanding about the medication? Could I share with you the reasons why the team is suggesting adding lithium to your current medication?	Lithium is a medication that has been used as a mood stabilizer for patients with bipolar disorder.	It could also be used to help patients with depression. How it works is by enhancing the effects of the antidepressants that you are currently on.
Discuss investigations prior to the commencement of lithium	Before we start lithium, we need you to do some basic blood investigations. These include a thyroid function test as well as a kidney function test.	In addition, we also like to recommend a heart tracing be done. Whilst you are on the medication, it is necessary for us to do routine blood tests to measure the lithium level. This enables us to know how much of the medication is in your blood. The normal ranges are between 0.4 and 1.0.	The blood tests (lithium levels) might be quite frequent initially, but once we have adjusted the medication to the right dose for you, we will repeat the test once every three months.
Describe side effects—short-term and long-term	Like all medication, lithium does have its side effects. The common side effects are thirst, passing more urine than usual, a bad metallic taste, and occasional tremors of the hands.	The long-term side effects might include that of weight gain. In a small percentage of patients, lithium does cause abnormalities in renal and thyroid functioning. Therefore, we will do regular blood tests to monitor this. I understand that you are very concerned about lithium and its effect on the kidneys. I'm sorry to learn of what has happened to your father. There are many other causes for renal disease, but I hear your concerns and will make sure we will monitor closely.	Other side effects might come on when the lithium levels are too high in the body. This might happen due to drug interactions and dehydration. If you are prescribed lithium, there are some medications, such as painkillers, water-losing tablets, high blood pressure medications, that you need to avoid as these could interact with lithium and raise the lithium levels in your body. If the lithium levels in the blood are high, you could have symptoms

(Continued)

(Continued)

			such as diarrhoea, vomiting, severe hand tremors, and maybe even confusion. Please come back to see us immediately.
Address other concerns	The time for response varies amongst individuals. Hopefully, the addition of lithium to your existing antidepressant will help you with your recurrent depressive episodes. It is not wise to stop the medication immediately once you feel that you're better. You should come back to us, and we could discuss more best to help you.	Lithium is not an addictive medication, and this means that you do not need to take increasing doses to get the same effect. We like you to inform your other doctors that you are on lithium as there are certain medications you cannot take.	As lithium might cause heart abnormalities in a foetus, please let us know if you have plans to start a family. It would be best if you considered contraceptive options whilst you are on lithium. We would not advise you to take lithium in combination with alcohol. I understand that I have given you quite a lot of information. Could I offer you a brochure to help you understand the medication further?

Common pitfalls:

a. Failure to engage the patient and discuss with her the rationale for the commencement of lithium as she is feeling quite hopeless about her multiple admissions.

b. Failure to acknowledge her concerns about renal failure and reassure her that it is not a common side effect and that routine monitoring would be done for her (should she be on lithium).

c. Failure to address adequately all her concerns.

d. Failure to warn her about contraceptives and need to inform the team should she have any intentions to start a family.

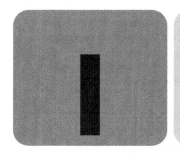

STATION 18
EXPLAIN
ELECTROCONVULSIVE
THERAPY

Information to candidates:

Name of patient: Mr Thomas

Mr Thomas saw the psychiatrist four months ago, and he was initially started on fluoxetine for his depressive symptoms. As he did not respond to the medication, the dose of fluoxetine was increased to 40 mg, and another antidepressant was added. He has been compliant and has been taking his medication. However, collaborative history from the wife indicates that his mood is still much the same, and he has not improved since the commencement of pharmacological therapy. The team has discussed his case, and the team consultant has decided that Mr Thomas might benefit from electroconvulsive therapy. You are the core trainee-3, and you have been tasked to provide Mr Thomas with more information about electroconvulsive therapy to enable him to come to an informed decision.

Task: Please explain to Mr Thomas the rationale for electroconvulsive therapy and address all his beliefs, concerns, and expectations.

Outline of station:

You are Mr Thomas, and you started seeing the psychiatrist around four months ago, after being made redundant at work for depression. He initially started you on fluoxetine 20 mg, but it did not seem to help you much with your mood. Hence, the medication (fluoxetine) was increased to 40 mg after eight weeks. The increased dose of medication did not do you any good, and your mood remained low. An additional antidepressant was added on. Your condition has not improved even with the addition of another alternative antidepressant. Your wife feels the same way as well.

You wonder whether the new treatment, now recommended by the team, would really help you with your condition. If the core trainee is empathetic enough towards your condition, you will ask him to explain more about the procedure. You have heard that the procedure was barbaric in nature based on media reports. You have concerns pertaining to the potential benefits, efficacy, side effects profile, and you also wish to know more about whether the procedure could be stopped once you have made some improvement.

CASC Construct Table:

The CASC Construct Table is formatted such that candidates would be able adequately to cover both the range and depth of the assessment required in this station.

DOI: 10.1201/9781003313113-18

Approach: Be prepared that the patient might be reluctant to try any new interventions as he has been on several antidepressants previously but with no success. You must demonstrate empathy towards the patient and explain the rationale for recommending the current treatment.

Starting off: "Hello, I am Dr Melvyn, one of the psychiatrists from the mental health unit. The team wants me to discuss with you the option of starting you on electroconvulsive therapy. Is that all right with you?"

Clarification of the rationale for ECT	Could I check with you whether you have heard anything about ECT before? Thanks for sharing your understanding with me. I'd like to explain to you more about ECT. Is that okay?	ECT refers to electroconvulsive therapy. It is one of the commonly used therapies, which is recommended by NICE, to help people with severe depression who have not benefitted from antidepressants.	ECT has been used for mania and schizophrenia as well. In your case, my understanding is that the doctors have tried you on several antidepressants (2), and your mood has not improved significantly. Hence, we'd like to help you with your condition using ECT.
Explanation of ECT Procedure	Before listing you for the treatment, we need to do some basic bloodwork and possibly a tracing of your heart rhythm to make sure you are medically fit to undergo the procedure.	The treatment is usually given two times in a week. During the procedure, the anaesthetist will give you some medication to help you relax and go to sleep. In addition, he will also give you some oxygen to breathe.	When you are relaxed and asleep, we will administer a small amount of electric current using electrodes to your brain. This will induce a short period of fit. It is believed that the induced fit would alter the brain chemical levels responsible for regulating your mood, appetite, and sleep.
Clarifications of concerns relating to ECT	As I have mentioned, ECT is a commonly used treatment modality in various psychiatric units. It is not a barbaric form of treatment as portrayed in the media.	The risk associated with ECT is very low. The mortality rate from ECT is 1 in 10,000 patients who have received ECT. The risk of death is rare and similar in percentages to that of a normal surgery.	
Explain benefits and potential side effects	The reasons why we are keen for you to consider ECT are that you have tried 2 previous antidepressants, but	As with all modalities of treatment, ECT has known side effects. Immediately after the procedure, some patients complain of	More commonly, you might lose memory over trivial events before the ECT. Rarely, you may encounter problems with the formation of new

	they have not worked for you. We hope that ECT would work for you and enable you to recover quicker. Switching and adjusting medication for your depressive symptoms might take a longer period. Previous research has shown that ECT is helpful in 80% of individuals. In addition, ECT can also help reduce the risk of suicide.	muscular aches and headaches. We could help with this by giving you painkillers. ECT does have effects on your memories— old memories and the formation of new memories. Some patients experience memory difficulties after ECT, but most of them usually improve with time.	memories six months after the ECT procedure. This latter side effect is more common among older patients. We usually also start ECT with the lowest energy level to minimize its effect on memory. At times, to minimize memory issues, unilateral ECT is conducted (electrodes placed on the right side of the brain). The number of sessions is usually 6–12, depending on your condition, done three times per week.
Discuss consent issues and address other concerns	As with all procedures, we are required to ask you to sign a consent form for the procedure. Signing the consent form does not mean that you are mandated to undergo all the sessions you have signed for. You could withdraw your consent at any point in time.	Do you have any other queries pertaining to ECT? I understand that I have given you quite a lot of information. Could I offer you a brochure about ECT?	Please feel free to book an appointment to see us again to discuss further about ECT or other alternative therapies.

Common pitfalls:

a. Failure to reassure the patient that ECT is not a barbaric form of treatment and build rapport with the patient to continue explaining more about ECT.

b. Overemphasis on the explanation of the side effects of ECT and failure to bring across the point as to why the team wishes the patient to consider ECT.

c. Failure to address the patient's concern about side effects of ECT and possible remedies: such as using unilateral electrode placement.

Information to candidates:

Name of patient: Mr Johnson

Mr Timothy Johnson is a 21-year-old university student who has been admitted to the inpatient mental health unit as his hostel mates noted that he was experiencing auditory hallucinations over the past two months. The team has done the necessary bloodwork and radiological imaging; thus far, they are all normal. The team consultant feels that Mr Johnson has a diagnosis of first-episode psychosis and has started him on olanzapine to help him with his unusual experiences. His mother, Sarah, is very frustrated to learn that he has been diagnosed with first-episode psychosis. She has come down today expecting to know more about the diagnosis and prognosis of his condition.

Task: Please explain to Mrs Sarah Johnson the diagnosis and discuss with her the prognosis of her son's condition.

Outline of station:

You are Mr Johnson, and you have been sectioned for admission to the local mental health unit following experiencing two months of auditory hallucinations. The team doctors have told you that you have first-episode psychosis, and they have started you on a medication known as olanzapine. You feel better since they have commenced the medication, though you feel quite sedated on taking it. You are keen to get well as soon as possible and be discharged home soon.

Your mother, Mrs Sarah Johnson, is here, and she appears to be very agitated about learning from the nurses that her son has first-episode psychosis. She has researched much about the condition online, and she is very concerned that her son has been diagnosed with this condition. She demands to know the prognosis of her son's condition, and she also wants to know whether her son can get back to university life.

CASC Construct Table:

The CASC Construct Table is formatted such that candidates would be able adequately to cover both the range and depth of the assessment required in this station.

DOI: 10.1201/9781003313113-19

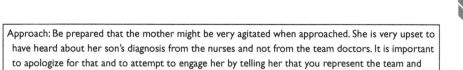

Approach: Be prepared that the mother might be very agitated when approached. She is very upset to have heard about her son's diagnosis from the nurses and not from the team doctors. It is important to apologize for that and to attempt to engage her by telling her that you represent the team and you're here to explain and address all her concerns.

Starting off: "Hello, I am Dr Melvyn, one of the psychiatrists from the mental health unit. I understand you are here today as you have concerns about your son, Timothy. Could we have a chat about it?"

Clarification of diagnosis	I must apologize that you learned about your son's diagnosis from the nurses. It should have come from the doctors. Please let me speak to the team to ascertain why this has happened. I understand how concerned you are with regards to your son's condition. I'm hoping that we could make use of this interview to address all your questions, as we would like to work collaboratively with you to get your son better.	I'm sorry to tell you that the team feels that your son has a condition known as schizophrenia. Have you heard about this before? Schizophrenia is a relatively common mental health condition that affects approximately 1% of the population. Patients usually develop symptoms around the age of 20.	The common symptoms of schizophrenia include positive and negative symptoms. By positive symptoms, I am referring to the presence of unusual experiences, such as hearing voices, seeing images, or having strange feelings in their body. By negative symptoms, I am referring to symptoms such as low mood, low energy levels, and lack of interest. Are you following me so far?
Explain aetiological causes	I need to reassure you that you are not to be blamed for your son's current condition.	Research has demonstrated that there are multiple causes for schizophrenia. Some individuals might be predisposed, as they have a positive family history; other causes include infections during pregnancy, delivery complications, the usage of street drugs, and the presence of certain genes that might predispose individuals to have schizophrenia if they use cannabis. A chemical imbalance in the brain involving the neurotransmitter dopamine results in the core symptoms of schizophrenia.	Unfortunately, unlike other medical conditions, there are no specific tests that we can do to diagnose someone with schizophrenia.
Explain management plans	Usually, when someone is acutely ill, we might need to treat them in our inpatient unit. There are various ways	We have started your son on a medication known as an antipsychotic. It would help to regulate his brain chemical and control the symptoms.	Apart from medication, there are other forms of treatment that are helpful.

(Continued)

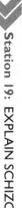

(Continued)

	in which we could help them, by using medication and other non-medication methods.	Like all medication, antipsychotics do have their own side effects as well. The common side effects include sleepiness, weight gain, restlessness, and muscle stiffness.	We could make use of talking therapy, like cognitive behavioural therapy, to help them deal with their distressing symptoms. Psychoeducation is essential in allowing the individual and his caregivers to understand more about the illness. Other forms of therapy might include family therapy, art therapy, rehabilitation, and courses and training to help individuals reintegrate back into their employment.
Address concerns and expectations	Your son would need to take the medication for a period of time. You could help us by supervising him to ensure that he takes his medication. If he stops the medication, there is a high chance that those symptoms which have been bothering him might reappear again.	Despite what is commonly portrayed in the media, patients with schizophrenia are rarely dangerous.	I am hopeful that, with the medication he is on, and with your assistance in supervising his medication, he should eventually return to his previous work/ studies. I have shared quite a lot of information. Could I offer you a leaflet to bring home?

Common pitfalls:

a. Failure to apologize to the mother at the start of the interview.
b. Failure to engage the mother (it is important to tell the mother that you are here to address all her concerns so that you can work collaboratively with her to get her son better).
c. Failure to alleviate guilt (it is important to explain that there are multiple aetiological factors that might predispose an individual towards developing psychosis).
d. Failure to discuss the psychosocial approaches regarding the management of the condition.
e. Failure to inform the mother regarding various types of psychosocial interventions (just mentioning CBT alone).
f. Failure to offer the mother a prognosis of her son's condition.

STATION 20
EXPLAIN
PSYCHOSOCIAL
INTERVENTIONS FOR
SCHIZOPHRENIA

Information to candidates:

Name of patient: Mr Wicks

Mr James Wicks is a patient with a chronic history of schizophrenia. He is currently here for a follow-up with outpatient services. He was last admitted to the inpatient unit about one month ago for a relapse of his schizophrenia. He has been trialled on several antipsychotic medications, but they have not been effective in keeping him well. Some of his prior relapses are due to his non-compliance with his medication. Since his recent discharge, a community psychiatric nurse has been assigned to follow up with him. During a recent home visitation, the community psychiatric nurse noted that his family members tend to be hostile when communicating with him. His father has accompanied Mr Wicks for his routine outpatient follow-up appointment today. He is keen to know your management plans to help prevent relapses of his son's condition and how he could best help as a caregiver.

Task: Please speak to James's father. Please address all his concerns and expectations.

Outline of station:

You are James's father, Mr Wicks. You are accompanying your son to his medical appointment today. You're concerned about your son's deteriorating mental health condition (frequent relapses). You feel that the team has not provided him with the best possible care. You are upset that your son has been discharged with the same medication after his last admission. You do not feel that the medication keeps him well. You are appreciative that the team has arranged for a community psychiatric nurse to follow up with his care. You like to know how you could, as a caregiver, best support your son in keeping him well. You like to discuss with the psychiatrist how your communication styles within your family might have an impact on your son.

CASC Construct Table:

The CASC Construct Table is formatted so that candidates can adequately cover both the range and depth of the assessment required in this station.

DOI: 10.1201/9781003313113-20

Approach: Be prepared that the father might be irritable when discussing his son's condition. It is important to demonstrate empathy and to listen to and understand his concerns.

Starting off: "Hello, I am Dr Melvyn, one of the psychiatrists from the mental health unit. I understand you are here today as you have concerns about your son. Could we have a chat?"

Understanding his concerns	Given his multiple relapses, I understand that you're quite distressed about your son's condition. I like to use this opportunity to clarify any concerns and doubts you have. I hope that you appreciate that we are concerned too and would like to work collaboratively with you to help James.	What is your understanding of your son's condition? Do you know that he has been diagnosed with schizophrenia? What do you understand about schizophrenia? Are you concerned about his multiple relapses? How has his condition affected your relationship with him? Has it also had an impact on his relationships with other family members? I understand from the community psychiatric nurse that you've some concerns about his medication. Would you be able to share more with us?	I understand that this has been a difficult time for you. I am glad you have shared this with us as we would like to help you and advise you on how best you could care for your son.
Clarify recent admission and management plans	I hope I could clarify what happened regarding the previous admission. When James was admitted a month ago, it was a voluntary admission.	As it was a voluntary admission, he is not legally bound to remain in the hospital to receive continued treatment. While in the hospital, we offered him a new medication, but unfortunately, he declined and told us he is only willing to take the previous medications. We did not have an opportunity to make use of the Mental Health Act for James, as he improved when he remained in the hospital. Hence, we needed to go with his choice.	However, we understand that James has suffered from relapses quite frequently. Hence, the team of doctors decided that the community psychiatric nurse should visit James more frequently to check on his mental state and ensure his compliance to medication. There are multiple reasons why there has been frequent deterioration in his mental state. It might be that he has not been compliant with the prescribed medication or that the depot medication that he is on is not effective for him. At times, when individuals abuse other substances/drugs, they might cause a deterioration in their mental state.

Explain proposed management—admission and pharmacological interventions	I understand how difficult things have been for you. We hope we can work collaboratively to help your son, James. For now, we will ask our community psychiatric nurse to visit James more regularly to check on his mental state. Should there be any deterioration, we might need to invoke the Mental Health Act for him to be admitted.	If he is to be admitted, the team might want to consider him on an alternative medicine known as clozapine. This medication is usually reserved for patients with schizophrenia that has not responded to adequate doses of previous antipsychotics. If we are thinking about starting clozapine, we will need to register him with the CPMS (clozapine patient monitoring system), and we will start him with the lowest dose.	Clozapine, like other medication, does have its side effects as well. The common side effects include that of sedation, decreased blood pressure, and hyper-salivation. I understand that you are very concerned that James might not agree to inpatient admission. We will make sure we do frequent visitations and try to explain to him why he needs an inpatient stay. If he strongly declines an inpatient admission, we might need to admit him under the Mental Health Act. Unfortunately, even though you are his caregiver, the act does not allow you to give consent for involuntary admission. Thanks for sharing with us his drinking issues. It is important for him not to drink if he is started on new medication. If he is admitted, we will assess his drinking issues in further detail and help James with it.
Explain proposed management—interventions targeting expressed emotions and other psychological interventions	The community psychiatric nurse has highlighted that the way you and your family members communicate with James might be a trigger for his relapses. Some family members have high expressed emotion. High expressed emotion includes	I would like to recommend family intervention and communication training in view of your concerns regarding communications within the family. In addition to medication, I'd like to refer James for cognitive behavioural therapy. Through this therapy, he will learn how to monitor his own thoughts, feelings, and behaviours, and he will be taught ways to cope with his psychotic symptoms.	I would also like James to be assessed by our occupational therapist to see if he could be commenced on art therapy. Art therapy would help him express himself and relate better to others. If James is keen to pursue future employment, we could explore other options, such as that pre-vocational training or programmes that would support his integration back to work.

(Continued)

(Continued)

	hostility (where the patient/his condition gets blamed for problems in the family), emotional over-involvement (over-protectiveness within the family, excessive use of praise or blame), and critical comments (complaints about the patient). Have there been instances in which such comments have been made?		In addition, I like him to follow up with his GP for routine screening as he is on antipsychotic medication. Do you have any other concerns?

Common pitfalls:

a. Failure to deal with an angry parent.
b. Failure to address all his concerns and expectations (lack of range and depth of information covered in the station).
c. Failure to identify and exclude factors that might account for treatment resistance.
d. Failure to address high expressed emotions is one factor leading to his relapsing.
e. Failure to discuss appropriate intervention strategies for high expressed emotions.
f. Failure to explain other psychosocial interventions.

STATION 21
EXPLAIN BIPOLAR
AFFECTIVE DISORDER

Information to candidates:

Name of patient: Ms Lee

Ms Lee is a 26-year-old administrator who was diagnosed with depression one year ago and has been on an antidepressant, citalopram, for the past year. She has been informally admitted to the mental health unit, as her family members realize that she has had a massive change in her mood state. She was noted to be very irritable and, at times, very elated and had spent huge amounts of money on investments and even harboured unusual ideations that she was the royal family's chosen one. She has since been admitted to the inpatient mental health unit and has been there for two weeks. Ms Lee is aware that the team stopped her antidepressants and then started to treat her with antipsychotic medication to help her stabilize her mood. She has been informed that she has a bipolar affective disorder. She learnt from her treatment team that they are considering her on a mood stabilizer. She has heard about mood stabilizers like sodium valproate before, and she is concerned about the risks associated with their use. She is keen to know more about her condition, the side effects of common mood stabilizers like sodium valproate, and the alternative medicines that could be considered. She is also concerned about her risk of relapses.

Task: Please speak to Ms Lee to explain her diagnosis, clarify her doubts about her medication, and address all her concerns and expectations about her condition. You do not need to perform a mental state examination.

Outline of station:

Much of the history is in the introductory notes for this station. You are Ms Lee, and this is the first time you have had a manic episode after having been treated for what seemed to be depression one year ago. You understand from the team that you have been diagnosed with bipolar affective disorder but have limited understanding about it and wish to know more. You are keen to know the reasons why you are predisposed to having it. You have heard about mood stabilizers like sodium valproate before and are concerned about its potential side effects. You wish to know more about alternative treatment. You also wish to know more about the prognosis of your condition as it will affect your chances of getting back to work.

DOI: 10.1201/9781003313113-21

CASC Construct Table:

The CASC Construct Table is formatted such that candidates would be able adequately to cover both the range and depth of the assessment required in this station.

Starting off: "Hello, I am Dr Melvyn, one of the psychiatrists from the mental health unit. I understand from the team that you have some concerns. Could we have a chat?"			
Explain bipolar affective disorder	I understand that the team informed you that you have bipolar affective disorder. Have you heard about this before? Bipolar affective disorder is a common mental health disorder that affects, on average, every 1 in 100 persons. It is called bipolar disorder as there are two poles in this disorder—mania and depression.	When an individual is in the manic phase, they would feel very elated in mood and be full of energy despite not getting much rest. They might be spending more money than usual and might be less inhibited in terms of their social activities. They tend to speak very rapidly and might have a lot of plans.	In contrast, when a patient is in the depressive phase, they would have low mood with a reduction in interest. There might also be difficulties with sleep and appetite. At the extremes, some people do have suicidal ideations, and some might act on their ideations.
Clarify causes	Bipolar affective disorder usually starts prior to the age of 30.	I hear that you are concerned as to what causes you to have this disorder. The exact cause is unknown, and research has demonstrated that several factors might predispose someone to have this disorder.	If you have a family history of a psychiatric disorder, you have a higher chance of acquiring it. Chemical imbalances and environmental stressors might also be contributing factors as well.
Explain medication	Are you aware of how bipolar disorder is being treated? Since the time that you have been admitted, the team has decided to stop your antidepressant. You should continue to avoid using any antidepressant medication as it might worsen your condition.	The team has started you on antipsychotic medication, that of olanzapine. Antipsychotic medication like olanzapine could help in stabilizing your mood in the acute phase.	The team is now considering if you should be commenced on a mood stabilizer. Mood stabilizers which are commonly used include that of lithium and sodium valproate.

Clarify concerns regarding mood stabilizer (valproate)	Have you heard of mood stabilizers before? I understand that you are concerned about being on sodium valproate. Please let me explain further and clarify any doubts that you might have. Sodium valproate is a medication that is commonly used for individuals with fits of epilepsy. However, it could also be used as a mood stabilizer for patients who are in the manic phase. It has been used since the 1990s to treat individuals with bipolar disorder. It works on a chemical in the brain called GABA.	While valproate is an effective medication, it could harm the fetus if you're pregnant. Valproate could result in the following birth defects: (a) spina bifida (bones of the spine not joining up properly); (b) cleft lip and palate; (c) other abnormalities involving the limbs, heart, or kidneys. This happens in 10% of women who take valproate during pregnancy. Developmentally, it is also likely that children would have developmental delays and are more predisposed to conditions like autism and attention deficit hyperactivity disorder.	Hence, given these concerns, we will carefully consider if you should be commenced on sodium valproate. If you are to take valproate, it is important that you use effective contraception whilst on treatment. Other medication could be considered that are likely to result in less harm to the baby. These are common side effects if you are commenced on sodium valproate. They include sleepiness, weight gain, increased appetite, nausea, and hair loss. A small minority of individuals on the medication might have abnormal liver function test, and some females do experience other side effects relating to their menstrual cycle. In particular, the use of valproate could result in a condition called polycystic ovarian syndrome.

(Continued)

(Continued)

Explain alternatives	Other medication could help in your condition. Antipsychotics like olanzapine will help you in your condition. Alternatives to olanzapine include quetiapine, risperidone, and haloperidol.	Other alternatives for mood stabilizers include lithium, carbamazepine, and lamotrigine. Have you heard of any of these before? Given that this is your first episode of mania, we could maintain you on an antipsychotic medication for now. If you have a second episode, it is pertinent that we consider other mood stabilizers.	Apart from medication, psychological therapy is also important. It is important that you keep track of your mood. Therapies like cognitive behavioural therapy could help with your condition.
Address concerns	I am hopeful that if you comply with the medication, you should be able to return to work. It is also important to be regular with your appointments.	Before we end this interview, I am hoping I could also provide you with some leaflets about bipolar disorder and how to help yourself. The leaflets would tell you how to cope with your condition and recognize the early relapse signs.	

It is important not to keep loading the patient with medical information, resulting in a "monologue." Remember to ask about what the patient has experienced in terms of her symptoms and relate them to the characteristics of the condition (this can help to make the discussion more relevant and easier to absorb for the patient). Furthermore, do pause intermittently and check for understanding.

Common pitfalls:

a. Failure to address all concerns and expectations (lack of range and depth of information covered in the station).
b. Failure to recognize the risk of prescribing sodium valproate to women of childbearing age.
c. Failure to explain other psychosocial interventions.

STATION 22
LITHIUM USAGE
DURING PREGNANCY

Information to candidates:

Name of patient: Ms Catrell

Ms Catrell is a 28-year-old female who has been diagnosed with bipolar affective disorder since the age of 25. She has been sectioned for admission to the inpatient unit on three occasions following manic relapses. The team has since decided to start her on a mood stabilizer known as lithium carbonate. She has been taking lithium carbonate 400 mg for the last year and has not had a relapse since. She has just got married and is keen to start a family. She has been on a contraceptive, as the team consultant who saw her previously advised.

Task: Please speak to Ms Catrell to address all her concerns and expectations. It is unnecessary to take a history or perform a mental state examination.

Outline of station:

Much of the history is in the introductory notes for this station. You are Ms Catrell, and you have been diagnosed with bipolar affective disorder since the age of 25. You used to suffer from frequent manic relapses, and it was only recently that the team decided to start you on this mood stabilizer, known as lithium carbonate. You have been compliant with the medication and have been on lithium carbonate 400 mg daily. Your serum lithium levels are in the therapeutic range. It might be because of the team's decision to keep you on lithium that has kept you off a relapse for the past year. The team consultant has previously advised you to use contraceptives since you are on lithium. You have just got married and are now keen to start a family with your husband. You wish to discuss more the usage of lithium in pregnancy. You do not wish the lithium to be stopped abruptly as you have witnessed its efficacy over the past year. You hope that the doctor will be able to address all your questions and concerns and deal with all your expectations.

CASC Construct Table:

The CASC Construct Table is formatted such that candidates would be able adequately to cover both the range and depth of the assessment required in this station.

DOI: 10.1201/9781003313113-22

Approach: Be gentle when exploring the benefits and risks of being on lithium in pregnancy. The patient might be quite reluctant to be off her mood stabilizer as it has kept her well for the past year. Starting off: "Hello, I am Dr Melvyn, one of the psychiatrists from the mental health unit. I understand that you are here today as you have some concerns about your medication. Could we have a chat?"			
Clarifications about mood stabilizer	I understand that you have some concerns pertaining to the lithium carbonate that you have been on. Could you tell me more?	Thanks for sharing, and congratulations on getting married. From what you have shared, it seems that lithium carbonate has kept you well over the past one year, such that you have had no relapse.	I understand that you are keen to start a family. Has anyone told you about the issues pertaining to the usage of lithium in pregnancy?
Explain risk of lithium in pregnancy	I'm sorry, but I must inform you that mood stabilizers like lithium are contraindicated in pregnancy. If you are on lithium for stabilization of your mood, we will generally recommend you stop the medication. There are other alternatives to keep you well during pregnancy.	However, given that you have been stable on lithium previously, an abrupt stoppage of the medication might cause a relapse.	Also, I do understand that pregnancy is very stressful. The stress you faced during pregnancy might precipitate a relapse. Hence, we must have this discussion today to work out how best we could help you plan.
Explain risk after pregnancy	Some individuals who are without their usual mood stabilizers do have relapses.	For a minority of individuals who relapse when they are not on their usual medication, they might find themselves having difficulties with caring for their infant.	
Explain the risk to the infant	In addition, we need to stress that lithium is contraindicated in pregnancy as it has been known to cause a heart defect known as the "Ebstein anomaly" in the fetus. Ebstein anomaly is a rare heart defect that's present at birth. In this condition, the heart valve is in the wrong position, and the valve's leaflets are malformed. As a result, the valve does not work properly. Blood might leak back through the valve, making your heart work less efficiently.	As you have a history of bipolar affective disorder, there is also a heightened chance that your infant might acquire the disorder.	For mothers with a relapse during pregnancy, their children's wellbeing and development might be affected.

Advise on alternative management options	I understand that you are very concerned about the withdrawal of lithium prior to you planning for a pregnancy, and I am aware that you are also concerned about having a relapse.	I suggest that I try to adjust your lithium and stop it gradually before we advise you to stop your contraception. I will keep you free from lithium during pregnancy. However, given that you have a history of multiple relapses, we could make use of alternative medication, like older-generation antipsychotics, to keep your mood stable during pregnancy	Once you have delivered, I recommend you recommence on lithium as soon as possible. However, as you have been recommenced on lithium, it is not advisable for you to breast-feed. Therefore, I will recommend that you give your infant bottles instead. I know that we have discussed a lot today. Please allow me to give you a leaflet on lithium in pregnancy.

Common pitfalls:

a. Failure to cover the range and depth of the station adequately. (You need to explore the risk of withdrawing lithium for the mother during pregnancy and consider the risk after pregnancy as well as the risk to the infant.)
b. Failure to discuss alternative medication during pregnancy to avoid a relapse of her underlying bipolar affective disorder.
c. Failure to highlight that breast-feeding is contraindicated if the mother is on lithium

It is important not to appear paternalistic about treatment options and insist on stopping lithium or not breast-feeding, etc. It would be better if you could provide a balanced opinion about all possible medical options and let the patient decide after having some time for consideration.

Information to candidates:

Name of patient: Mr Josephson

Mr Josephson is a 30-year-old male who has been diagnosed with depression since 2011. He was initially treated with fluvoxamine 50 mg in 2011, and his symptoms were remitted after one year into treatment. The antidepressant was thus stopped. Recently, he was told to leave his workplace, and over the past three months, he has what seemed to be a relapse as he has been having persistent low mood associated with a marked loss of interest. He came back to the mental health service, and his original antidepressant was restarted. However, his symptoms did not improve, and hence, the dose was further increased. After six weeks on the increased dose of the previous antidepressant, the psychiatrist felt that he had not responded to the treatment and has switched him over to venlafaxine 150 mg for now.

Task: Please speak to Mr Josephson and discuss the treatment options available, as he is keen to recover as soon as possible. Please do not take a history or perform a mental state examination.

Outline of station:

Much of the history is in the introductory notes for this station. You are Mr Josephson, and you have been diagnosed with depression since 2011. You were started on fluvoxamine 50 mg previously, and you recovered from that episode. However, three months ago, you were told to leave your job as a teacher. Since then, you have been experiencing a low mood associated with a marked loss of interest. Your psychiatrist has tried to adjust the dose of the antidepressant you have been on previously, but you have not noted many changes after six weeks on the higher dose of the medication. Your psychiatrist thus decided to switch you over to venlafaxine 150 mg, hoping that it would do you good. Unfortunately, nothing much has improved. You are keen to get well soon, and you are keen to hear from the doctor what alternatives are available that could help you get better soon.

CASC Construct Table:

The CASC Construct Table is formatted such that candidates would be able adequately to cover both the range and depth of the assessment required in this station.

DOI: 10.1201/9781003313113-23

Starting off: "Hello, I am Dr Melvyn, one of the psychiatrists from the mental health unit. I understand you are here today as you have concerns about your condition. Could we have a chat?"			
Explore reasons leading to poor response	Could I understand from you more about your condition? When were you diagnosed with depression? Could I check with you whether you have other medical conditions? Do you have any underlying hormone disorders, such as low thyroid function? Are you on any long-term medication for your other medical conditions? For example, are you on long-term blood pressure medication?	I know that it has been a difficult time for you. How have you been coping? Have you used any alcohol or drugs to help you cope?	Are you taking the antidepressant daily? Have there been any side effects with the medication? Apart from the stressor you shared, have there been any other problems, such as finances or in your relationships?
Discuss potential alternatives and explore alternatives for his current condition	Could you tell me more about the medication you have tried thus far? I understand how difficult it must have been for you. What we could do now is we could potentially increase the dose of the venlafaxine that you have been on and observe your mood.	Prior to us increasing the dose of the venlafaxine, could I check with you whether you have any family history of any medical problems? Is there a history of hypertension? If you have pre-existing hypertension, the increased dose of venlafaxine may worsen hypertension. We might need to also perform some basic investigations prior to the increment of the medication.	At times, a combination of medication and talking therapy might be more helpful. Have you heard of talking therapy before? Talking therapies like cognitive behavioural therapies could help you with your current condition. Cognitive therapy could help change your cognitive biases, while behavioural therapy helps with activity scheduling.

(Continued)

(Continued)

Explain the concept of treatment-resistant depression	If, after adjusting the dose of your second antidepressant to an appropriate dose and you still have not shown any response, it does seem to us that you have treatment-resistant depression. Have you heard of treatment-resistant depression before?	Treatment-resistant depression usually occurs when an individual has not shown an adequate response to an adequate dose of two different antidepressants that have been tried for an adequate duration of time.	There are still many other alternatives if your depression is indeed treatment resistant. We could consider enhancing the effects of your existing antidepressant by using either another antidepressant or by using other medication.
Clarify the use of ECT	ECT and repetitive transcranial magnetic stimulation (rTMS) might be one the other alternatives if you do not show much response to antidepressants.	I understand that I have shared quite a lot of information with you today. Do you have any questions for me?	

Common pitfalls:

a. Failure to identify reasons leading to poor response.
b. Failure to discuss alternatives prior to recommending ECT or rTMS. (In this case, the existing antidepressant medication dose could be adjusted first, and augmentation strategies could be tried first prior to ECT.)

You need to know the various augmentation techniques in managing treatment-resistant disorders.

STATION 24
OBSESSIVE-COMPULSIVE DISORDER (HISTORY TAKING)

Information to candidates:

Name of patient: Sarah Green

A 35-year-old housewife has been referred by her general practitioner (GP) to your service for further assessment. She has given birth to her son, Jordan, 6 weeks ago. She has been increasingly troubled by fears that Jordan might be infected with the new variant of the H1N1 influenza virus. Owing to her distressing worries, she has been finding it increasingly difficult to care for her young baby.

Task: Take a history to arrive at a potential diagnosis.

Outline of station:

You are Ms Sarah Green and have just delivered your son, Jordan, six weeks ago. This is your first pregnancy. You used to have obsessive–compulsive disorder (OCD), which was first diagnosed by your GP when you were at the age of 25. You have been treated with clomipramine previously, but this medication was stopped because of excessive sedation you have had from the medication. You were switched over to sertraline and have been on a stable dose. This medication was stopped around 1 year ago, when your symptoms had markedly improved after a combination treatment with both medication (sertraline) and psychotherapy (exposure and response prevention). After the birth of your child, it seemed like those symptoms had reappeared. You are troubled by recurrent ruminations pertaining to fears of contamination. This has resulted in you having to sterilize the milk bottles of your infant a fixed number of times (eight times). In addition, you have begun to have obsessional doubts and realize that you need to check things, such as switches, eight times. Your mood has been affected by your symptoms, but you still struggle to get by each day. Your family has been largely supportive, and your husband has taken over much of the care of Jordan, as you have been finding it increasingly difficult to care for your child and to ensure that he is getting his feeds on time.

CASC Construct Table:

The CASC Construct Table is formatted such that candidates would be able adequately to cover both the range and depth of the assessment required in this station.

DOI: 10.1201/9781003313113-24

Starting off: "Hello, I am Dr Melvyn. I have received some information from your GP regarding the difficulties that you have been having. Would you mind telling me more?"			
Core OCD Symptoms — DIRT: Doubts, impulses, ruminations, and thoughts	**Origin of thoughts** Can you tell me more about those worries that you have been having? How long have you had them? Did anything happen before the onset of these worries/obsessions?	**Exploration of other obsessional thoughts** Are you also concerned about needing to arrange things in a special way? Do you also have thoughts, images, or doubts that keep coming to your mind?	**Exploration of other compulsions** Do you find yourself needing to check very frequently? Do you find yourself needing to count in a particular pattern/manner?
	Do those thoughts come from within your mind, or are they imposed by outside persons or influences? **Nature of thoughts** Are those thoughts that you have repetitive in nature? Are they bothering you consistently even though you do not wish to have them?	Do you have constant doubts and find yourself needing to question? Do you have any aggressive or unwanted thoughts? Can you share more? **Exploration of compulsions** Tell me more about how you have been dealing with those obsessional thoughts? Have you been cleaning more often? Is there a particular number of times you need to clean? (Magic number) How do you feel after performing the rituals?	Do you find yourself needing to arrange items in a particular way? Do you find yourself repeating a particular word or phrase? Do you find yourself needing to perform other rituals to prevent something bad from happening?
Current functioning	**Impact of illness** Could you tell me how these rituals have impacted your life?	Have they affected other areas of your life, such as your relationships etc.?	
Other symptoms	**Assessment for depressive symptoms** How has your mood been? Are you still interested in things you used to enjoy?	How have you been sleeping? How has your appetite been? Have these mood symptoms come on before your OCD symptoms?	Are there other worries that you have been having?

Coping mechanisms	It has been a difficult time for you. Have you used alcohol to help you get through these difficult times? Have you used any other drugs to help you cope with this difficult time?	*(If there is still time, the candidate should check for tic disorder, PANDAS, and other OCD spectrum disorders such as hoarding, pulling of hairs when under stress.)* Can I check if you have any other medical conditions? Do you have any history of tic disorder?	Are you able to recall if you had a fever when you were much younger, prior to the onset of these OCD symptoms? Have you been hoarding items at home? Have you observed yourself to be pulling your hair when you're stressed?

Common pitfalls:

  a. Failure to cover the range and depth of the OCD symptoms.
  b. Failure to assess the impact of the symptoms.

Assess for the characteristic of "obsession" and "compulsion" in the interview and explore other themes and types of obsessions and compulsion, respectively.

Information to candidates:

Name of patient: Mr Leung

Mr Leung has been previously referred by his GP to the local mental health service to seek treatment for his OCD. He has been previously referred to a psychologist to receive psychological treatment. After undergoing several sessions of psychological treatment, his symptoms have not improved. He has been recommended to try fluoxetine, an antidepressant to help him with his symptoms. You are the core trainee in charge of your service's anxiety disorder clinic, and your consultant has asked you to speak to him.

Task: Please speak to Mr Leung and explain the recommended medication. Please also address all his concerns and expectations.

Outline of station:

You are Mr Leung, and you have been having increased fears of contamination ever since a laboratory accident happened six months ago, when there was a chemical leakage. Ever since then, you realized that due to your constant fears, you always needed to wash your hands multiple times to reduce the fears. You do not have other comorbid anxiety or depressive symptoms. This has affected your life significantly as you are always late for appointments and contemplating quitting your lab job. You have seen the psychiatrist previously, and he recommended that you see a psychologist to receive what is commonly known as cognitive behavioural therapy. You have been consistent with the sessions arranged, but you have not had much improvement. During the last outpatient review with the consultant, he recommended that you try an antidepressant known as fluoxetine. You are having doubts about being on medication. You have searched online and are concerned about the antidepressant being addictive. You are glad to be able to speak to someone who could address all your concerns and expectations.

CASC Construct Table:

The CASC Construct Table is formatted such that candidates would be able adequately to cover both the range and depth of the assessment required in this station.

DOI: 10.1201/9781003313113-25

Starting off: "Hello, I am Dr Melvyn. I have received some information from the consultant you have been seeing. I understand you have some concerns. Could we have a chat about this?"			
Explain and clarify indications for SSRIs	I understand from the consultant that he has previously recommended you for psychological treatment? How have the sessions been for you? I'm sorry to hear that the sessions have not helped you with your symptoms.	OCD is a very common mental health disorder that could be treated using psychological treatment, medication, or both. Have you heard about any medication that might be helpful for OCD?	The medication that we feel will help you with your condition belongs to the group of antidepressants called SSRIs, or selective serotonin reuptake inhibitors. It helps in the regulation of the chemical known as serotonin, which has been implicated for both OCD and depression. The dosage of the medication used for OCD is usually higher for OCD as compared to the dosage used for depression. SSRIs such as fluvoxamine, fluoxetine, paroxetine, sertraline are commonly used.
Explain the effectiveness and side effects of SSRIs	The success rates for patients with OCD who are on medication are around 50 to 80%.	Like all medication, SSRIs do have some side effects. The common side effects include that of nausea, gastric discomfort, headaches, and dizziness. These side effects are usually related to the dosages of the medication that are prescribed. We will monitor you closely with regard to the side effects and adjust the dosages accordingly.	We usually need you to continue the medication for some time till your symptoms are in control.

(Continued)

(Continued)

Address concerns	I need to clarify that antidepressants are not addictive in nature. Sometimes, we do prescribe sleeping pills or anxiolytics to help you when you first start on the antidepressant. Only those anxiolytics are addictive.	The chance of having a relapse is high if you were to discontinue the medication abruptly. We recommend that you discuss with us if you have any concerns pertaining to the medication, and we will advise you accordingly.	If SSRIs still do not help you with your symptoms, we could try switching you over to another medication called clomipramine or, for treatment-resistant cases, adding an antipsychotic to enhance the efficacy of the antidepressant.
Address the need for inpatient treatment	I am hopeful that the commencement of an antidepressant will greatly help you with your symptoms.	An inpatient stay might not be necessary at this stage as your symptoms are not so severe and life-threatening.	In addition, we have also not tried all the recognized forms of therapy.

Common pitfall:

a. Overemphasizing on the side effects of the medication and forgetting to tell the patient more about the clinical efficacy of the medication.

STATION 26
POST-TRAUMATIC
STRESS DISORDER

Information to candidates:

Name of patient: Mr Jones

Mr Jones has been referred by his local GP to the mental health service. He was deployed for military service in Iraq and was sent back prematurely as his commanders noted that he was not able to cope with his work demands. The referral letter from the GP stated that Mr Jones currently has no intentions to return to continue his job. The letter also states that there was an occasion on which Mr Jones needed to seek medical help in Iraq after being involved in an intense crossfire with the enemy forces.

Task: Please speak to Mr Jones with the aim of clarifying the history that the GP has provided. Please also perform a mental state examination with the aim of coming to a diagnosis. It is also pertinent during the clinical interview to rule out other psychiatric disorders.

Outline of station:

You are Mr Jones, and you have been previously deployed for military duties in Iraq. You served and functioned in your duties without any issues for six months. Unfortunately, you and your colleagues were then involved in an intense crossfire with the enemy forces. You witnessed how your best friend succumbed to that intense crossfire. This has affected you much, and you broke down that very night. You find yourself crying continuously, and your commanders asked the local medical doctor to see you. He gave you some pills to calm you down. However, since then, you have been having a lot of difficulties. You find yourself not being able to perform in your job. Your colleagues have commented that your mood seems more irritable lately. Your concentration has been poor, and you have been bothered by flashbacks and nightmares of the incident. You have been finding yourself getting startled very easily. It has been a tough time for you, but you have not resorted to coping with using any alcohol or any street drugs. You are desperate for help.

CASC Construct Table:

The CASC Construct Table is formatted such that candidates would be able adequately to cover both the range and depth of the assessment required in this station.

DOI: 10.1201/9781003313113-26

Starting off: "Hello, I am Dr Melvyn. I have received some information from your GP. I understand that you have been undergoing a very difficult time. Could we have a chat about this?"			
Clarification of the incident/event	Would you mind sharing with me more about what has happened? Could you tell me, when did this incident take place? At that time, did you really think that you could have died? Any physical injuries that you have sustained? Any head injuries?	I'm sorry to hear about the incident. Could you tell me who was involved? Do you know what happened to your colleague? Any survivor guilt?	It has indeed been a difficult time for you. How did you feel immediately after the incident?
Elicit core symptoms of PTSD—intrusions	How have things been since you returned?	Are there times when you get flashbacks of the incident? Or times when you feel that you are reliving the incident again? Could you tell me more?	How has your sleep been? Have there been any nightmares that have been bothering you?
Elicit core symptoms of PTSD—hyper-arousal	How has your mood been? Do you find yourself more irritable than usual?	Have there been times when you feel easily startled? Could you tell me more?	How has your concentration been? What about your memory?
Elicit core symptoms of PTSD—avoidance	I understand that you have since been back to the United Kingdom. Do you have thoughts about returning to active duties abroad?'	After the incident, did you go back to the place where it occurred? Any avoidance?	
Elicit core symptoms of PTSD—emotional numbing	How do you feel if you come across news or events like what you have experienced?	Do you find it tough to have normal experiences? Or to talk about how you feel?	Have you ever felt like the people around you (derealization) or yourself (depersonalization) are not real?

Assess for compensation/legal involvement and rule out other comorbidities	Are you currently involved in any legal suits or compensation claims in view of the incident? Any history of experiencing traumatic events? Any history of mental illness?	Do you find yourself having an interest in things you previously liked to do? How has your appetite been? Sometimes when people undergo stressful experiences, they do have unusual experiences. Does that sound like you?	Are there times to which you feel very anxious or have had worries about everyday events? I'm sorry to hear that this has been such a distressing experience for you. Have you used any alcohol or any other substances to help you cope?

Common pitfalls:

a. Failure to empathize with the patient adequately, and hence, failure to elicit the necessary information about the incident.

b. Failure to cover the range and the depth of the symptoms of PTSD.

c. Failure to ask and assess for compensation and other legal issues.

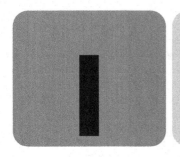

Information to candidates:

Name of patient: Mr Joel

Mr Joel has been missing from home for the past two days. He was found wandering in a shopping centre by the police, and he was brought into the emergency services by them. The medical team has done the necessary lab work, and everything thus far has been normal. You are the core trainee on call, and you have been asked to assess Mr Joel.

Task: Please speak to Mr Joel and perform a detailed cognitive assessment. Please do not take any history or perform a mental state examination.

Outline of station:

You are Mr Joel, and you wandered out of your house two days ago. You cannot remember the way back home since then. Your memory has been failing you for the past year, and you have been having a lot of difficulties lately due to your poor memory. You do not have hearing or visual impairment. You are willing to cooperate and perform the tasks that the core trainee asks you to perform.

CASC Construct Table:

The CASC Construct Table is formatted such that candidates would be able adequately to cover both the range and depth of the assessment required in this station.

Starting off: "Hello, I am Dr Melvyn. I understand that the police have brought you into the emergency services. I need to ask you some questions to test your memory. Is that all right?" *This station has been modified as the candidate may be asked to conduct an MMSE virtually. The adaptations made to perform MMSE virtually are highlighted within this station.*			
Assess for orientation	Before we begin, could I check whether you have any visual or hearing impairments? Could you see and hear me clearly?	Do you know where we are now? What level are we on? Which part of the county is this? What is the greater country that we are in?	Do you know what time it is now? Do you know what year this is? Can you tell me what season, month, and day and date today?
Assess for registration	I would like you to remember three objects, to which I will ask you to repeat immediately and five minutes later.	The three objects I'd like you to remember are "apple," "table," and "penny."	Can you repeat the three objects that I have told you?

DOI: 10.1201/9781003313113-27

Assess for attention and calculation	Could I trouble you to spell the word "world" for you?	Could you please spell the word "world" backwards for me?	(If the patient is unable to spell, assessment could be done using calculation/numbers instead.)
Assess for recall, naming, repetition, comprehension	Could you tell me the three objects that I asked you to remember earlier?	Could you name these objects for me? (Show the patient a pen and a watch.)	Could you please repeat this phrase: "Not, if, and, or buts?" Please listen to my instructions and follow my instructions. I'd like you to take this piece of paper with your right hand, fold it into half, and place it on the floor. (*Adaptations for online CASC:* Show me your right index finger, then use the right index finger to touch the nose, and then use the right index finger to touch the left shoulder.)
Assess for reading, writing, and copying	(Write **Close your eyes** on a piece of paper, assuming the patient has a piece of paper.) Could you please read this sentence and do what it says?	Could you help me write a complete sentence with a subject and verb?	(Draw two intersecting pentagons.) Could you please help me to copy this figure?

Common pitfalls:

a. Failure to ask the patient whether he has visual or hearing impairment prior to the start of the assessment.

b. Failure to remember all the steps in the MMSE and perform a complete MMSE.

c. Failure to make adaptations to the assessment of the three-step commands for virtual CASC.

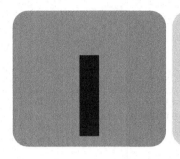

STATION 28
FRONTAL LOBE
ASSESSMENT

Information to candidates:

Name of patient: Mr Greene

Mr Greene has had personality changes after a head injury, which he suffered two years ago. His wife has accompanied him today, and they want some help from your specialized mental health service.

Task: Please speak to Mr Greene and perform a detailed cognitive assessment, looking for features suggestive of frontal lobe dysfunction. Please do not take a history or perform a mental state examination.

Outline of station:

You are Mr Greene, and you suffered a head injury following a fight at the local pub around two years ago. Since then, your wife has complained that you are no longer the person she once knew. She claimed that you have been more irritable than usual. She also claimed that your memory is not as good as it was before. This you alluded to as you realized you can no longer function in your finance job and have since left the company you have been working for the past 20 years. You are finally agreeable to an assessment by a psychiatrist today after much persuasion by your wife. You agree to cooperate with whatever tests the psychiatrists want you to perform.

CASC Construct Table:

The CASC Construct Table is formatted such that candidates would be able adequately to cover both the range and depth of the assessment required in this station.

Starting off: "Hello, I am Dr Melvyn, one of the psychiatrists from the mental health service. Thanks for coming to see us today. Will you be all right for me to ask you to do some memory tests?"			
Verbal fluency assessment	Before we start, can I ask whether you have any visual or hearing impairments? Please do feel free to stop me at any time if you do not understand me.	I would like you to say as many words as possible starting with the letter F in one minute, without using any names of people. Could we begin?	Alternatively, I would like you to say as many animals as you can within one minute. Could we begin?

DOI: 10.1201/9781003313113-28

Abstract thinking assessment	Could you tell me your understanding of this proverb, "A stitch in time saves nine."	Could you tell me about the similarities between an apple and an orange? (Alternatively, use a table and chair as example.)	Could you tell me what the average height of an Englishman is? Could you tell me the approximate distance (in miles) between London and Manchester?
Assessment of coordinated movements	Please have a look at this diagram (alternate sequence of squares and triangles). Could you copy this diagram for me?	I like you to place your index finger on the table. Please raise your index finger once when you feel a single tap, and do not raise it when you feel two taps. Could we try this?	Now, I am going to reverse the rule. Please do not raise your index finger when you feel a single tap; raise it when you feel two taps. Could we try this?
Assessment for response inhibition	I am going to show you a sequence of hand movements. (To demonstrate to the patient the specific sequence of a fist, then placing the edge of the palm and then a flat palm on the table.)	I'd like you to follow my sequence of hand actions.	Do you think you could show me the sequence?
Primitive reflexes	Now, I am going to test some of your reflexes.	I would need to place my hands and gently tap between your eyebrows. Are you fine with this?	Next, I will need to gently stroke your palm. Are you fine with this? I need to use the spatula to gently tap on your lips. Are you fine with this? Thanks for your cooperation.

Adaptations for Online CASC: For the alternative sequence test, you might need to show the patient an example of the alternating sequence of squares and triangles and get him to prepare a piece of paper to copy it. It might not be possible to perform the go-no-go test and the test of primitive reflexes. For the assessment of response inhibition, one could adapt it and use a clipboard for demonstration.

Common pitfalls:

a. Failure to ask the patient whether they have visual or hearing impairment prior to the start of the assessment.
b. Failure to remember all the steps in the frontal lobe assessment battery.
c. Failure to ask the patient for permission prior to testing for primitive reflexes.

Information to candidates:

Name of patient: Ms Molloy

Ms Molloy is a 25-year-old university student who has been admitted to the accident and emergency department following an overdose on 20 tablets of medication. The medical doctors have done the necessary, and currently, she is medically stable. However, the medical consultant has requested for her to be seen by a psychiatrist in view of the recent overdose.

Task: Please speak to Ms Molloy and obtain a further history of the recent overdose. Please also perform a relevant suicide risk assessment.

Outline of station:

You are Ms Molloy, a 25-year-old university student. You have been found by your hostel-mate in your hostel room, unconscious and brought into the hospital. You have just overdosed on 20 tablets of a combination of medicines. Your recent stressor was that you failed a major university examination. This is your first failure in life. You felt disappointed and felt that there was no longer a meaning to live on as your opportunities to find your dream job are compromised. You made a deliberate plan and attempted to end your life, and you are upset that you have been found.

CASC Construct Table:

The CASC Construct Table is formatted such that candidates would be able to cover adequately both the range and depth of the assessment required in this station.

Starting off: "Hello, I am Dr Melvyn, one of the psychiatrists from the mental health unit. I have some information regarding what happened this morning. Could we have a chat?"			
Assess suicide plan and intent	I have some limited information about what happened this morning. It must have been a very difficult time for you. Could you tell me more about why you took the 20 tablets of medication? Were you troubled by any significant life events recently?	Was the overdose planned? Have you considered or contemplated it for long? How did you manage to have access to those medicines? What did you think would happen if you took all of them?	Have you thought and hoped that you would take your own life by taking an overdose?

DOI: 10.1201/9781003313113-29

Assess the circumstances of the suicide attempt	Where did you take the medication? Was anyone else there, or were you likely to have been found? Did you lock the door or take any precautions to avoid discovery?	Did you take other medication besides these tablets? Did you mix the medication with alcohol? Did you harm yourself by other means?	Did you leave a suicidal note? Did you send an SMS or email to say goodbye to your partner or family members?
Assess events after the suicide attempt	How did you manage to come to the accident and emergency department? Did someone else discover you?	Did the overdose lead to any physical discomfort? Did you have a period of blackout?	How do you feel about it now? Do you regret your suicide attempt? Would you do it again?
Assess for the presence of risk factors or protective factors	Have you attempted suicide previously? If yes, when was it? How many times have you done so? Did you try other methods like hanging, stabbing yourself, jumping from heights, or drowning?	Do you have any history of any mental health disorder, such as depression? Are you suffering from any other illnesses? Any family history of mental illness/disorder?	We have spoken quite a lot about the overdose and some of your stressors. I understand that it has been a difficult time for you. Are there things in life you are looking forward to?

Common pitfall:

a. Failure to cover the range and depth of the information required for this station.

STATION 30
SUICIDE RISK
ASSESSMENT (PATIENT
MANAGEMENT)

Information to candidates:

Name: Dr Thomson

Ms Molloy is a 25-year-old university student who has been admitted to the accident and emergency department following an overdose on 20 tablets of medication. The medical doctors have done the necessary, and currently, she is medically stable. The medical consultant has requested for her to be seen by a psychiatrist in view of the recent overdose. You have been tasked to speak to her to get a history about the suicide attempt, as well as to perform a current suicide risk assessment. In this station, the on-call consultant has heard about this case and is awaiting your call to discuss with him more details about the case.

Task: Please speak to Dr Thomson, the on-call consultant, to further discuss the circumstances surrounding the overdose and to discuss the management of the case, given the risks involved.

Outline of station:

You are Dr Thomson, the on-call consultant. You have learnt about this case and understand that your core trainee has been tasked to assess the patient. You are expecting a consultation by your core trainee. You wish to know more about the circumstances surrounding the overdose. You expect that the core trainee has performed a comprehensive suicidal risk assessment, and you wish to know the current risk. You will then proceed to discuss with the core trainee more about the specific management plans.

CASC Construct Table:

The CASC Construct Table is formatted such that candidates would be able to cover adequately both the range and depth of the assessment required in this station.

Starting off: "Hello, I am Dr Melvyn, one of the core trainees. Could I discuss a case with you?"			
Brief formulation of the case	Dr Thomson, I have been asked to see a 25-year-old university student in the Emergency Department. She was found and taken to the hospital by her friends following an overdose on a variety of 20 medications in total.	I have spoken to her and the current stressor contributing to the overdose seemed to be of a recent failure in her academics. There are no other stressors that I could identify.	The medical team doctors have treated her for the overdose and have asked us for an evaluation.

DOI: 10.1201/9781003313113-30

Evaluation of the suicidal intent and the seriousness of the attempt	I understand from her that she has made plans for the overdose and have accumulated the medicines over a total duration of three days. She left a suicide note for her parents and tried to conceal the attempt by locking the doors and making sure her friends were not at home	She was fully aware of the seriousness of the attempt and wanted to end it off entirely by taking the pills. She is currently expressing regrets with regards to her being rescued by her friends.	She has not taken other adjunctive medication and has not consumed alcohol together with the medicines.
Current risk assessment	When I spoke to her, she was still vocalizing that she had thoughts of suicide. She claimed that there was nothing to stop her from attempting something more lethal, and she was determined to make it a success.	She does not have any past psychiatric disorders, and she does not have a family history of any psychiatric conditions. This is the first time she has overdosed on medication.	My current suicide risk assessment would place her at high risk given the circumstances of the recent overdose, as well as her current suicide ideations.
Management plans	Given the current risk, I suggest that she be admitted to the inpatient unit for further observation and stabilization. In the short term, we need to observe her closely and place her on the necessary suicide caution.	We might consider starting an antidepressant if her mood is clinically low, but only when she is medically stable and her labs are normal.	I feel that she would benefit from further engagement with a psychologist, who could teach her some coping strategies as well as engage her in some form of therapy. We might need to consider other supports she could engage in whilst at school. Do you have any questions for me?

Common pitfall:

a. Failure to cover the range and depth of the information required for this station.

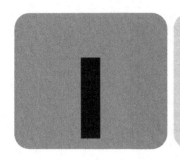

STATION 31
GRIEF REACTION

Information to candidates:

Name of patient: Mrs Davis

Mrs Davis, a 60-year-old female, has been referred by her GP, as her GP has noted that her mood has been low for the past couple of months since her husband's passage. The GP is concerned that she might be depressed and hopes that she could benefit from being seen and being managed by a mental health specialist.

Task: Please speak to Mrs Davis to take a history of her presenting symptoms to establish a diagnosis.

Outline of station:

You are Mrs Davis, a 60-year-old female, and your GP has referred you to a psychiatrist for your mood symptoms. Your mood has been low since the sudden passage of your husband six months ago. He died from a heart attack and was totally unexpected. You do not have any dependents, and hence, you are currently staying alone in your home. You did manage to attend your late husband's funeral. Previously, you were feeling emotions of denial, anger, and had bargained about why God has been so unfair towards you. Recently, in the past month or so, you have noticed that your mood has been low, and you have been more emotional. You do not have any interest and have been confining yourself at home. You have been having poor appetite and sleep. You do not have any perceptual disturbances, and you do not have any suicidal ideations.

CASC Construct Table:

The CASC Construct Table is formatted such that candidates would be able to cover adequately both the range and depth of the assessment required in this station.

DOI: 10.1201/9781003313113-31

Starting off: "Hello, I am Dr Melvyn, one of the psychiatrists from the mental health unit. I understand that your GP has referred you to see us. Could we have a chat today?"			
History of presenting complaint/ nature of husband's death	I received some information from your GP. I'm sorry to hear of all that has happened recently. I understand that it must have been a very difficult time for you. It would be helpful if I could understand a bit more about your husband's recent passage. Would you mind sharing with me more about what happened?	I'm sorry to hear that. You mentioned that it was unexpected and sudden. Were you with him when it happened? What happened thereafter? Could you tell me how long ago this was?	Was there any form of closure for you? Did you manage to attend the wake? How were you coping then? Have you been to his burial place since? How was your relationship with your husband?
Exploration of her current stage of grief/ assessment for comorbid depressive symptoms	Sometimes, when people experience the loss of their loved ones, they do experience a whole range of emotions. You have lost someone significant, and recently you have been feeling quite emotional about it.	Have you ever felt angry? Do you blame anyone for causing the death? Were there times in life to when you started to bargain, wishing that it were you instead of your husband?	How have you been feeling in your mood recently? Do you feel that your mood is low and you have been very emotional? Are you able to enjoy and partake in activities to which you used to enjoy previously? What are your energy levels like? How is your sleep? What about your appetite? Are you able to concentrate and focus on things you wish to do? Do you think you have come to terms with your recent loss?
Exploration for symptoms suggestive of atypical grief	Some individuals who have lost their loved ones tend to leave their loved ones' belongings as if they were still around. Does that sound like you?	Are there times to which you felt as if you could hear your husband still?	Do you feel responsible for his death? Are you feeling guilty about anything? Have you felt that life has lost its meaning? Do you feel that life is not worth living anymore? Have you ever have had plans to take your own life?

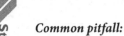

Common pitfall:

a. Failure to cover the range and depth of the information required for this station.

It is important to ascertain the circumstances of the loss and the relationship between the deceased and the patient. For younger patients, you will also need to check for dependents, which may potentially be a risk factor for abnormal grief as one may not be able to express the grief fully.

STATION 32
BODY DYSMORPHIC DISORDER

Information to candidates:

Name of patient: Mr Rahman

You have been tasked to speak to Mr Rahman, a 30-year-old gentleman. He is a taxi driver, and he has been referred by his GP to see you in the mental health service. You gathered from the referral memo that he has visited his GP recently, requesting a specialist referral to a plastic surgeon. The GP has stated that Mr Rahman has been insistent on a referral to a plastic surgeon for correction of a deformity of his nose. The GP has not identified anything abnormal; hence, he is hoping that you could evaluate him prior to him being referred and possibly undergoing any corrective surgery.

Task: Please speak to Mr Rahman to better understand his current problems. Please take sufficient history to formulate a clinical diagnosis.

Outline of station:

You are Mr Rahman, and you are a taxi driver. You have been troubled by your nose problem since you were a teenager. You always remember how your peers tease you and bully you in school. You firmly believe that there is something abnormal about your nose, in terms of the way it is shaped. Because of this deformity, even though you have managed to graduate from university with a business degree, you are not able to work in an office job. You have resorted to working as a taxi driver as you do not need to face people that much. As a result of your nose problem, you do not have many friends and have yet to be in a relationship. You cannot help checking in the rear-view mirror at times due to your concerns about your nose deformity. You avoid going out to events, and there has been a time to when you needed to resort to some special way of grooming to hide the deformity. You are keen for immediate help. You do not understand why you must see the psychiatrist when all you want is for the GP to refer you to the plastic surgeon for definitive surgery to correct the defect. You have watched some videos online, and you feel that if the doctors are not going to help you, there might be a chance you might take things into your own hands and correct it yourself. You do not have a past psychiatric history of note.

CASC Construct Table:

The CASC Construct Table is formatted such that candidates would be able adequately to cover both the range and depth of the assessment required in this station.

DOI: 10.1201/9781003313113-32

Starting off: "Hello, I am Dr Melvyn, one of the psychiatrists from the mental health unit. I understand that you have been referred by your GP. Could we have a chat?"		
History of presenting complaint	I understand that you have been to your GP recently to request a referral to a plastic surgeon. Could I understand more about that? I'm sorry to hear about the distress that you have had. It is not uncommon for us to speak to patients prior to them undergoing a procedure.	You mentioned that you had been troubled by your nose deformity. Could I understand from you when this all first started? Was it just recently? When did you first notice that you have had such a problem? Apart from you noticing it, what have others said?	It seemed like this has been a chronic problem that has troubled you for many years. Do you feel increasingly more concerned about it recently? Was there any trigger that caused you to feel this way recently? It seems to me that you are very concerned about the shape of your nose. Do you have any other concerns about any other body parts?
Assessment of the strength of beliefs and challenging beliefs	You mentioned that you feel that there is something wrong with your nose. However, it seemed to me that other people had not commented so.	Could it be that there is really nothing wrong with your nose? How convinced are you that there is something wrong with your nose?	If the plastic surgeon tells you that there is really nothing wrong with your nose and that no surgery is required, would you be amenable to his suggestion?
Impact of illness	I'm sorry to hear that this has been a problem that has been bothering you for many years. I understand that you are keen to have a quick fix of your problem. Before we get about to discuss more how best we could help you with your problem, can I understand how this problem has affected you over the years?	Has it affected your work? Has it affected your relationships with your family members? Has it affected your relationships with your peers? Do you tend to avoid certain situations due to the defect of your nose?	Are you very concerned about the deformity of your nose that you would spend a lot of time looking at it, say, in a mirror? How much time do you spend daily? How frequently do you check? Have you resorted to camouflaging your deformity in the event you have a social gathering to attend to?
Risk assessment	Are you so distressed by the nose issue that you have ever felt that life has no meaning for you? Have you contemplated or entertained thoughts of suicide before?	What are your plans if the surgeon is not willing to do the surgery for you?	Do you have any plans to correct the deformity yourself? Could you tell me more about what you have in mind with regard to what you might do to yourself?

Ruling out other comorbid psychiatric disorders	How has your mood been recently? Do you still have an interest in things you used to enjoy doing?	How has your sleep been? What about your appetite? Could you still function at work? Sometimes, when people undergo stressful experiences, they report having unusual experiences. Do you have similar experiences?	Have you seen a psychiatrist before? Is there anyone in the family who has a mental health history?

Common pitfalls:

a. Failure to cover the range and depth of the information required for this station.
b. Failure to ask for specific risk related to body dysmorphic disorder, such as self-operation.

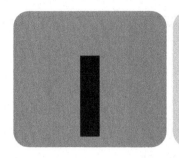

STATION 33
SLEEP DISORDERS—
INSOMNIA

Information to candidates:

Name of patient: Mr Foster

You have been asked to see Mr Foster. He has been referred by his GP for sleeping difficulties. He does not have any other chronic medical conditions, aside from hypertension.

Task: Please speak to Mr Foster and elicit a history to come to a potential diagnosis.

Outline of station:

You are Mr Foster and have visited your GP a couple of days ago, as you have been having difficulties with falling asleep. You do not have any other medical conditions apart from hypertension. You do not have a family history of mental health conditions and have not seen a psychiatrist before. You are married, but recently, there has been increasing stress due to relationship issues. You are employed now and are just coping with the job that you have been assigned. You have done routine blood investigations, and they are all normal. You will provide the psychiatrist with a copy of the results. Your GP has not prescribed you any medication but has advised you on sleep hygiene methods. You have tried them, but you are still having many difficulties with the initiation of sleep. You hope the psychiatrist can explain to you what is wrong with you and suggest a treatment for your condition.

CASC Construct Table:

The CASC Construct Table is formatted such that candidates would be able to cover adequately both the range and depth of the assessment required in this station.

DOI: 10.1201/9781003313113-33

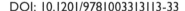

Starting off: "Hello, I am Dr Melvyn. I received some information from your GP. Can we have a chat about it?"			
Explore sleep issues and rule out medical causes	I understand from the memo from your GP that you have been having some difficulties with your sleep. I'm sorry to hear that, and I know that it must be difficult for you. Can you please tell me more about your problem? When did this first start?	Can you take me through a typical day of yours? Can you tell me more about your routine before bedtime? Do you have a problem with initiating sleep? Have you been waking up more than two times at night (and this waking up is not due to you needing to use the bathroom)? Have you found yourself waking up very early in the morning? Do you have nightmares at night? Has this been a problem for you previously? How has your sleep issues affected your daytime functioning?	Can you tell me if you have any physical or medical conditions that I need to know of? Do you have obstructive sleep apnoea (snoring)? Are you on any medication for your hypertension? What sort of work do you do? Does any shift work? Assess the patient's current sleep hygiene.
Explore current mental state	How has your mood been recently? Do you find yourself feeling low? How would you rate your mood currently? Is there variation in your mood in a day? Do you find yourself being able to enjoy things that you used to enjoy?	Apart from your sleep difficulties, have you been experiencing issues with your appetite as well? How do you find your energy levels to be? Are you able to concentrate on doing things that you used to enjoy?	Can you tell me if there is anything that is stressful for you now? Can you tell me more? Have you ever felt that life is meaningless? Have you ever entertained thoughts of ending your life? Have you ever had any strange experiences, such as hearing voices when no one is there?
Explore personal history	Have you seen a psychiatrist before? Can I ask if there is anyone in the family who has a mental health condition?	Do you use substances such as alcohol? What about drugs?	How would you describe yourself in terms of your personality?

(Continued)

(Continued)

Explain management plans	I understand that your GP has given some sleep hygiene advice previously. I'm sorry to learn that it did not seem to have helped you with your condition. Based on my assessment, your mood is not clinically depressed.	Thanks for sharing your difficulties with your sleep. It helps us better determine if you have initial, middle, or terminal insomnia. I would recommend that we try the sleep hygiene tips that we shared previously.	If these techniques do not work, we could consider starting you on a low dose of sleeping medication. We will aim to use these for a short time as I am concerned about their inherent addictive potential.
Address concerns and expectations	Do you have any questions for me?		

Common pitfalls:

a. Failure to cover the range and depth of the information required for this station.

b. Failure to assess sleep problems in depth (differentiating between initial, middle, and terminal insomnia).

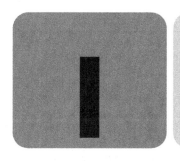

Information to candidates:

Name of patient: Mr Charleson

You have been tasked to assess Mr Charleson. He has been admitted to the medical ward as he has had two prior episodes of vomiting out blood. The medical consultant wishes to schedule him for an urgent endoscopy to find out the cause of the bleeding. The team has noted that he has had a history of schizophrenia. They are concerned about whether he is fit to sign the pre-operation consent forms. They have thus called in psychiatrists to assess this capacity to provide consent.

Task: Please speak to Mr Charleson and determine whether he can provide consent for the endoscopy that the medical team has scheduled him for.

Outline of station:

You are Mr Charleson, and you have been admitted to the medical ward. You have had two episodes in which you vomited out fresh blood. The medical team has seen you and advised you to undergo further evaluation, including an endoscopy evaluation. You have a rough idea of the procedure that is involved. The team has informed you of the potential complications as well. You have decided not to go ahead as you feel strongly that the surgeons might attempt to implant another chip in you.

CASC Construct Table:

The CASC Construct Table is formatted such that candidates would be able to cover adequately both the range and depth of the assessment required in this station.

Starting off: "Hello, I am Dr Melvyn. I received some information from the medical doctors who have seen you. They have requested that I come to quickly evaluate your condition. Can we have a chat about your condition?"			
History of current issues	I understand that you have been recently admitted to the hospital. Can you tell me more about what has been happening? How long have you had this problem for?	Is the problem getting worse? Can you tell me more?	What do you think is wrong with you?

(Continued)

DOI: 10.1201/9781003313113-34

(Continued)

Mental state evaluation	I understand that you have had a pre-existing mental health disorder. Can you tell me more about what condition you had? How long have you had this condition for? In the past, did you require any inpatient hospitalizations for your mental health condition? Are you currently on any medication for this condition? Have you been compliant with the dose of medication prescribed?	Over the past month, how has your mood been for you? Do you find yourself interested in things you previously used to enjoy? Are there any difficulties with your sleep or appetite? Have you had any unusual experiences? By that, I mean, do you hear voices or see anything unusual when you are alone?	Do you feel that there are others out there who are trying to harm you? Do you feel in control of your thought processes? Do you feel in control of your emotions and actions?
Assessment of mental capacity— ability to understand information	Can you share with me your understanding of what is wrong with you? What has the medical team told you with regard to your condition?	Did they tell you what they think might be the cause of the problem? Have they suggested that you need to be further evaluated?	Can you tell me more about your understanding of what they have told you with regard to further evaluation?
Assessment of mental capacity— ability to retain information	Did the medical doctors tell you what the advantages of endoscopy would be?	Did the medical doctors inform you about the risks associated with the procedure? Are there other life-threatening complications that they have informed you about?	Please allow me to explain why the medical doctors have recommended this procedure for you. Please also allow me to explain the potential complications that might arise from the procedure.
Assessment of mental capacity— ability to weigh information and come to a decision	Can you tell me once again why the doctors have made such a recommendation?	Can you tell me once again what complications the procedure is associated with?	Can you tell me your decision with regard to the procedure? Can you tell me the reasons why you are refusing the treatment? Is this your final decision?

Summarize and communicate that the best decision is not made	It seemed to me that you are worried about the procedure as you feel that the surgeons might implant a device within you. This is even though the team has clearly told you about the rationale for the procedure.	Unfortunately, this does not seem to be the best possible decision in the current situation. Please give me some time to discuss this with the rest of your medical team.	Would it be all right for me to return to speak to you about it again?

Common pitfall:

a. Failure to cover and summarize all four areas of capacity assessment (1. Understand and retain information about the procedure; 2. Patient understands the risk and benefits of the procedure; 3. Unable to weigh the pros and cons of the procedure, alternative procedure, or no treatment; 4. Communicate the decision clearly without the influence of psychopathology).

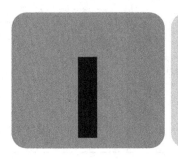

Information to candidates:

Name of patient: Mr Young

You have been tasked to speak to Mr Young. He has a history of vascular dementia and has been recently admitted to the hospital following a recurrent vascular infarct. The medical team has optimized his medication and arranged for him to undergo rehabilitation whilst he is in the hospital. The physiotherapist and occupational therapist have provided inputs about his social functioning, regarding which they have both recommended that he would need more social care support at home. The team has since recommended this option to Mr Young, but he has rejected the need for increased support. Given his history of dementia, the team has decided that the psychiatrist on call could help in the evaluation of his decision—and capacity-making ability.

Task: Please speak to Mr Young and determine whether he can make care arrangements, given that he has a background history of vascular dementia.

Outline of station:

You are the patient, Mr Young. You are 68 years old and diagnosed with vascular dementia five years ago. You needed inpatient hospitalization recently as you woke up one day to find that there was weakness on your left side. The medical doctors have diagnosed you with a recurrence of stroke. You have been asked to participate in rehabilitation programmes organized during the inpatient stay, which you have duly participated in. You were surprised when the team informed you that you would need further social care support when you're back home. You are not receptive towards having more people in your home.

CASC Construct Table:

The CASC Construct Table is formatted such that candidates would be able to cover adequately both the range and depth of the assessment required in this station.

DOI: 10.1201/9781003313113-35

Starting off: "Hello, I am Dr Melvyn. I received some information from the medical doctors who have seen you. They have requested that I come to do a quick evaluation of your condition. Can we have a chat about your condition?"			
Mental state examination	I understand that you have a pre-existing mental health disorder. Can you tell me more about what condition have you had? How long have you had this condition? In the past, did you require any inpatient hospitalizations for your mental health condition? Are you currently on any medication for this condition? Have you been compliant with the dose of medication prescribed?	Over the past month, how has your mood been for you? Do you find yourself having an interest in things that you previously used to enjoy? Are there any difficulties with your sleep or appetite? Have you had any unusual experiences? By that, I mean, do you hear voices or see anything unusual when you are alone?	Do you feel that there are others out there who are trying to harm you? Do you feel in control of your thought processes? Do you feel in control of your emotions and actions?
Assessment of ability to understand	I understand that you have been through the rehabilitation programme recommended by your doctors.	Have they told you their assessment of your condition? What do you know about your current condition?	
Assessment of ability to appreciate risks and benefits and to retaining information	Have the doctors told you their rationale for recommending social care support for you? Can you tell me more about what they have explained to you?	Have the doctors told you the dangers and risks involved if you do not have enhanced social care support?	I'd like to re-explain to you the advantages and the disadvantages of having increased social support.
Assessment of mental capacity— ability to weigh information and come to a decision	Can you tell me, once again, why the doctors have made such a recommendation?	Can you tell me, once again, what the risks might be if you do not have enhanced social care support?	Can you tell me your decision regarding this? Can you tell me the reasons why you are refusing the recommendations of your doctor?

(Continued)

(Continued)

Summarize and communicate that the best decision is not made	Thanks for speaking to me. Let me reassure you that the team is very concerned about your condition, and hence after careful evaluation, they have decided to make such a decision and recommendation.	The team is trying their best to help you with your condition whilst you are at home. I would like to re-discuss your case with the team of doctors caring for you again.	Would it be okay for me to return to speak to you about this again?

Common pitfall:

a. Failure to cover the range and depth of the information required for this station.

STATION 36
BREAKING BAD NEWS

Information to candidate:

Name of patient: Mr Penrose

Mr Penrose is an 80-year-old male who has been admitted to the psychiatric ward for an acute change in his mental state. Prior to this, he has been well and does not have any chronic medical conditions. He does not also have any underlying pre-existing psychiatric disorders. The team has evaluated his condition and has done some baseline blood investigations and a brain scan. All the blood investigations were within normal limits. The radiological investigation (a computed tomography scan of his brain) revealed a suspicious lesion. The neurologist has been called in for a further evaluation, and they feel that the lesion is most likely that of a meningioma. His daughter, who is his primary caregiver, is currently here and hopes to find out more about his condition.

Task: Please speak to his daughter and explain his current condition. Please address all her concerns and expectations.

Outline of station:

You are the daughter of Mr Penrose. You are his main caregiver and have been increasingly stressed about his condition. Your father has been healthy up until four months ago. You noticed that he has had personality changes. You are very concerned that last night he appeared to be very confused, and hence you decided to send him in for an extensive evaluation. You understand from the nursing staff that some baseline investigations have been done for your father. You hope to be able to speak to the team to understand more about his condition. You are devastated to learn that he has a brain lesion. You wish to know more about the prognosis of his condition. In addition, you hope to be able to obtain from the team their input regarding the possible treatment options. You hope to be able to bring him back home as soon as possible and will highlight this request to the team of doctors. You hope that the team of doctors can provide you with further information regarding the treatment plans and options.

CASC Construct Table:

The CASC Construct Table is formatted such that candidates would be able adequately to cover both the range and depth of the assessment required in this station.

DOI: 10.1201/9781003313113-36

Starting off: "Hello, I am Dr Melvyn. I understand that you wish to get some updates about your father's current condition. Can we have a chat about this?"			
Introduction and establishing what carer has known	I understand that it has been a challenging time for you. I hear that you wish to have an update about his current condition. Before that, can you please share with me more about what happened prior to the current admission?	Have you managed to visit your father before speaking to me? What do you understand about his current condition?	I wonder whether anyone has updated you regarding his current condition.
Gradually break the bad news	In view of the acute changes in his mental state, upon his admission, the team decided to perform a variety of tests, which included baseline blood tests and radiological scans. Thus far, the bloodwork that we have done seems to be fine.	I would like to share with you more about the results of the brain scan that we have done. Would it be all right for me to go on? Unfortunately, we noticed that there is a lesion in his brain when we did the scan. Are you alright with me going on?	(Allow the carer some time to accept the bad news.) What is your understanding of a brain lesion/brain tumour? A brain lesion/tumour is a tumour or a mass comprising of abnormal cells within the brain. It could either be cancerous or non-cancerous. The brain lesions might have accounted for the acute changes in his current mental state. I'm sorry that I need to be informing you of this news. Do you have any questions for me at the moment?
Discuss expectations and concerns	I understand that you are concerned with regard to the further treatment options. We have referred your father to the neurologist, who has since looked at the radiological scan.	Based on my understanding, there are several treatment options, which usually include surgery, radiotherapy, or even chemotherapy. However, I would not be in the best position to comment on which of these modalities of treatment are the best indicated currently as I am not a specialist in this area.	I hear your request that you wish to take him home. However, it might not be the best decision currently. We might need to run further investigations and tests to help in our diagnosis, and hence it would be better for him to stay in the hospital. Also, I understand that you have had a difficult time

		I'm hoping my neurology colleague will get back to us as soon as possible, and we will arrange a joint session to discuss treatment options.	managing him at home. We hope that we can help you in this aspect as well. We hear your concerns with regard to whether your father will be in pain. Please be assured that we will get our multidisciplinary team on board. We might give him some medication to help him with the pain that he is experiencing.
Summarize discussion	I know that we have given you a lot of information. Do you have any questions for me?	Do you need me to speak to anyone in the family?	

Common pitfalls:

a. Failure to cover the range and depth of the information required for this station.

b. Use of jargon and giving too much information without checking to see if the family member understands.

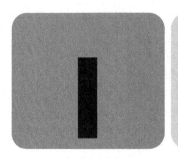

Information to candidates:

Name of patient: Mr Daniels

Mr Daniels, a 22-year-old university student, was admitted to the inpatient unit two days ago. He was admitted after his roommate found him behaving abnormally. Since admission, the team has acquired further history and diagnosed him with first-onset psychosis. Mr Daniels has a positive family history of mental health disorders. In addition, he has been using cannabis since the age of 15 years on a regular basis. The team has decided to start him on a course on antipsychotics as he was experiencing significant positive symptoms. However, he was noted to be spiking a high temperature this morning. The on-call core trainee who examined him found him to be rigid as well. The attending consultant suspects he might have developed neuroleptic malignant syndrome and has since transferred him to the intensive care unit. Mr Daniels's father is here now and is demanding to find out more about his son's condition.

Task: Please speak to Mr Daniels's father and address all his concerns and expectations. Please also provide him with an explanation of what has happened to his son.

Outline of station:

You are the father of Mr Daniels. You are very concerned that your son needed admission to the psychiatry unit and are devastated to know that he has first-episode psychosis. You hoped for the inpatient stay to be as short as possible and initially hoped that your son could get back to his baseline functioning as soon as possible. You are shocked to learn of the fact that your son is now being transferred over to the intensive care unit. You demand an explanation from the doctor in charge of him. You also wish to know the further prognosis of his condition. You also want to know what the plans are regarding the further management of his condition.

CASC Construct Table:

The CASC Construct Table is formatted such that candidates would be able to cover adequately both the range and depth of the assessment required in this station.

DOI: 10.1201/9781003313113-37

Starting off: "Hello, I am Dr Melvyn. I understand that you wish to get some updates about your son's condition. Can we have a chat?"			
Explain rationale for medication	I'm sorry to inform you that your son has been transferred to the medical intensive care unit. I understand that you're very concerned about his current condition. The team is also very concerned about his current condition.	As your son was experiencing florid symptoms of his psychosis, we needed to start him on a course of antipsychotics to help him with his symptoms. The team has commenced him on a low dose of antipsychotic (olanzapine).	This antipsychotic is commonly used for most patients, and most patients do not experience acute side effects after commencement.
Explain likely diagnosis— neuroleptic malignant syndrome and clinical features of the condition	It is very likely that your son has developed a condition known as neuroleptic malignant syndrome. Have you heard about this condition before?	Would it be all right for me to explain more about this condition? This is a rare condition that occurs in approximately every 1 in 100 individuals.	In this condition, it is not uncommon for individuals to have unstable vitals (heart rate and blood pressure). They might also spike a temperature. Clinically, on examination, these individuals are usually relatively rigid in their extremities. They might also have altered consciousness levels. It is a medical emergency, and hence we have transferred your son to the medical intensive care unit for more intensive monitoring.
Explain likely causes for NMS	The most likely cause of this condition is the antipsychotic medication that we have just commenced.	As said, this is an unpredictable and rare side effect of an antipsychotic medication.	Of course, there are other medical conditions that might present in the same way. We have done some basic laboratory investigations, and the findings are suggestive of neuroleptic malignant syndrome. The laboratory test showed that there was an increase in muscle breakdown. It is usually more common if patients are prescribed with the older generation of antipsychotics.

(Continued)

(Continued)

Explain further management	Given that neuroleptic malignant syndrome is considered to be a medical emergency, we have immediately arranged for a transfer to the medical intensive care unit. The medical team is also currently on board to help us with the acute management of your son's condition. We have since stopped the antipsychotics that we had recently introduced. He is also kept nil by mouth now to avoid choking.	We are monitoring his vitals very clearly and making sure that we are providing him with adequate hydration. Other cooling measures might also be considered. The medical team might consider the usage of other medication to help him with his condition. Such medication could help him to relax and moderate the levels of dopamine.	We will routinely do blood tests, and in particular, we will trend a blood test result known as creatinine phosphokinase. We will also monitor his blood counts, kidney, and liver functions. We will continue to monitor his condition, and we will provide you with regular updates.
Address concerns	Currently, the medical stability of your son's condition is of utmost importance.	We have since stopped the likely offending agent and have also reported that your son has an adverse reaction to that particular medication.	Once he is clinically more stable, we will try to re-challenge him with another antipsychotic medication, as it would be helpful for his symptoms.
Address complaints procedure	I would like to apologize for this. As said, NMS is a very rare condition, and it's difficult for us to know who would and would not acquire it.	I understand that you have some concerns which you would like to bring up to the hospital. Would you like me to guide you on the procedure?	I know that I have provided you with quite a lot of information today. Do you have any other questions for me?

Common pitfalls:

a. Failure to cover the range and depth of the information required for this station.
b. Use of jargon and giving too much information without checking the understanding of family members.
c. Failure to address parent's anger, giving a lecture on NMS, and not responding to parent's concerns.

It is essential to address the anger and frustration raised by the family member. Apologize for what the family has gone through but remember not to apologize for causing this (there is a huge difference in this!). It may be helpful to use reflective statements, especially at the start of the interview. For example, "I can see that you are very angry at this point. It is very understandable for you to experience this." Remember to address the family member's complaint and guide him to the appropriate channel. Do not push blame on anyone—it is essential to maintain collegiality towards colleagues.

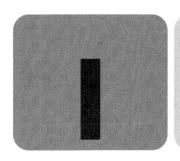

STATION 38
URINE DRUG TEST

Information to candidates:

Name of patient: Mr Wells

You have been tasked to speak to Mr Wells. He is a 30-year-old male with a history of paranoid schizophrenia and has just been admitted to the inpatient unit following a relapse of his condition. As he has been more settled in terms of his mental state, he was allowed on home leave. He has since returned from his home leave, and the nursing staff has contacted you. You are the on-call core trainee. During the interview, you noticed that Mr Wells appeared to be very distractible, and at times, he was observed to be mumbling to himself. You have discussed the case with your attending consultant, who recommended that you acquire a sample of the patient's urine, as he has been known to abuse cannabis previously as well.

Task: Please speak to Mr Wells and persuade him to give you a sample of his urine for testing. Please do not perform an MSE.

Outline of station:

You are the patient Mr Wells. You have a history of paranoid schizophrenia and have been admitted to the inpatient unit several times. You recently got admitted again as you have not been compliant with the medication that you were prescribed in the outpatient setting. Before admission, you harboured paranoid ideations, which led you to be cooped up at home as you were afraid that others out there might harm you. With the current inpatient treatment, you have gradually recovered and are currently better. You have been granted Section 17 home leave over the weekend. You are worried about returning home, so you spend your time at the nearby park instead. You met up with your friends, and they offered you some weed to try. You are reluctant to share this history as you know that it would lead to a longer stay in the hospital. Also, those paranoid ideations and auditory hallucinations have since returned as well.

CASC Construct Table:

The CASC Construct Table is formatted such that candidates would be able to cover adequately both the range and depth of the assessment required in this station.

DOI: 10.1201/9781003313113-38

111

Starting off: "Hello, I am Dr Melvyn. I understand that you have just been back from your home leave. Can we have a chat?"			
Explain indications for assessment	I understand that you have just been back from your home leave. The nurses are quite concerned about how you have been since you returned back and hence requested for me to see you. Would it be all right for me to have a chat with you?	I would like to understand from you how your home leave was. Would you be able to tell me more about it?	
Explain rules and regulations of Section 17 home leave	Is this the first time you are allowed on home leave? Are you able to tell me what your previous home leaves were like? What happened after you returned from your previous home leave?	One of the rules when our patients are under Section 17 home leave is that they might be asked to provide a sample of their urine after they return back to the ward. Had the team told you about this before you went on home leave?	We hope you can cooperate with us and provide the necessary sample. It would help us in the further management of your condition. We hope that you can get well and be discharged sooner.
Explore concerns about provision of urine sample	It seems to me that you are quite reluctant to provide us with your urine sample. Is there any reason why?	Did you spend your home leave at home? If not, where were you?	Can you tell me more about what happened? Was there a chance you were offered or used any drugs or alcohol during your scheduled home leave? We do need to know this as this will affect the medication we have prescribed, and it will also affect how we help you with regard to your current condition.
Exploration of possible psychotic symptoms	It seems to me that you have appeared to be very distracted throughout the interview. Is there anything bothering you?	Do you feel that there might be others out there who are plotting against you or who might harm you?	Do you have any strange experiences, such as hearing voices or seeing things that are not there? Do you feel in control of your thought processes? Do you feel in control of your emotions and actions?

Common pitfall:

a. Failure to cover the range and depth of the information required for this station.

For the patient in this station, it may be helpful to ask in an indirect and nonthreatening manner the circumstances of the home leave and his reasons for refusing a urine drug screen. Do not be overly fixated on insisting he go for the screening. It is important to address his concerns and alleviate his anxiety about the fear of being convicted if the drug screen comes back positive.

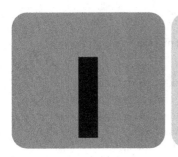

Information to candidates:

Name of patient: Mr Wells

You have been tasked to speak to the mother of Mr Wells. Mr Wells was diagnosed with schizophrenia at the age of 20 years, with the aetiology most likely due to chronic usage of cannabis since the age of 15 years. He has had multiple relapses that previously required inpatient admission and treatment under Section 2. Recently, he relapsed again due to his being non-compliant with medication, and he has since been in the ward for the past two months. The team has tried him on at least three typical and atypical antipsychotics and has commenced him on clozapine as he fulfils Kane's criteria for treatment-resistant schizophrenia. His mother is here today and is demanding to see a member of the team. She is distraught that her son would still require prolonged hospitalization and is also worried about the clozapine on which he has been started. She has read more about the medication (clozapine) on the Internet and has learnt of significant adverse effects. She wishes to bring him home today.

Task: Please speak to the mother of Mr Wells and attempt to de-escalate the situation and explain the rationale for her son being started on clozapine. Please address all her concerns and expectations.

Outline of station:

You are the mother of Mr Wells and are very upset with the management of the team. Your son has had multiple admissions to the hospital this year. You understand that the team has since started him on clozapine. You are upset that no one from the team has sought your perspective about it. You have done some research about it and know that it is associated with dangerous side effects. You do not want your son to have more medical problems in addition to his pre-existing psychiatric disorder and are upset with the rate of the progression of his condition. You do not find that it is helpful for him to remain in the hospital and wish to bring him home today. If the core trainee does not allow you or recommends you do so, you will ask for a discharge against medical advice.

CASC Construct Table:

The CASC Construct Table is formatted such that candidates would be able to cover adequately both the range and depth of the assessment required in this station.

DOI: 10.1201/9781003313113-39

Starting off: "Hello, I am Dr Melvyn. I understand that you have some concerns about your son. Can we have a chat?"			
Introduction, using empathetic statements to calm relative down	Thanks for coming today. I hope we can make use of this opportunity to clarify any concerns that you might have about your son's condition.	I'm sorry, and I do apologize for the fact that the doctors on the team did not inform you that your son has been commenced on clozapine.	Please let me speak to them to find out what has actually happened. However, I hope that I can try my best to address all your concerns. I understand that it has been a difficult time for you, given your son's multiple readmission and prolonged admission. I hope you understand that we are both trying our best to help your son with his psychiatric issues.
Explanation of rationale for clozapine	I hear your concerns about clozapine. Your son has had a trial of multiple antipsychotics, including the newer generation as well as the older generation of antipsychotics.	During this admission, we have adjusted the dosing of the medication accordingly, and we have tried administrating the maximum possible doses to your son. Unfortunately, it did not seem to help your son with his condition.	Given that, the team's opinion during our multidisciplinary meeting is that your son most likely has a condition known as treatment-resistant schizophrenia. Have you heard of this before? Can I take some time to explain to you what we mean and refer to as treatment-resistant schizophrenia? Treatment-resistant schizophrenia is diagnosed when a patient fails to respond to a trial of three antipsychotics of different classes, using an adequate dose of antipsychotics for an adequate duration.

(Continued)

(Continued)

Discuss side effects and monitoring procedures	I hear your concerns about the side effects of clozapine. Prior research has indeed shown that clozapine could cause agranulocytosis (a condition in which the body does not make enough white cells—neutrophils, so regular blood counts are necessary).	Hence, when your son was started on clozapine, we also organized regular blood tests for him. In the first 18 weeks, we are required to determine his full blood count on a weekly basis. In addition, we also monitor closely the other side effects associated with the medication, such as hyper-salivation.	We have started your son on the lowest dose of clozapine and have gradually increased the dose accordingly. We have done so to make sure that his body is able to gradually adapt to the effects of the medication.
Discuss management options	Despite the fact that we have already initiated your son on a course of clozapine, I'm sorry to inform his progress of recovery on the medication has been relatively slow.	Hence, we have kept him in the hospital so that we can adjust the dosing accordingly and monitor his condition more closely. I hear that you are concerned about him being admitted for so long, but our team is trying our best to help him using the new medication (clozapine).	In addition, one of the other concerns we have had was that, upon admission, we noticed that your son's LFTs were abnormal. Is there a possibility that he has been drinking prior to admission? Can you tell me more?
Advice against discharging against medical advice	I understand your concerns about the prolonged hospitalization. I hope we can better able to help your son during this admission so that his rates of relapse would be reduced. I hear that you wish to consider a discharge against medical advice. However, I hope that you can reconsider that.	One of our concerns about your son's condition lies with the fact that he might potentially be using alcohol. It is not recommended for him to be using alcohol when he is also using clozapine. We might need to refer him to the dual diagnosis unit to help him should your son have an alcohol problem as well.	I hear that you might want to raise a complaint against the team and the hospital. If I could help, I could direct you to the appropriate procedure. Do you have any other concerns that you would like to discuss today?

Common pitfall:

a. Failure to cover the range and depth of the information required for this station.

TOPIC II
GERIATRIC PSYCHIATRY

STATION 40
GERIATRIC PSYCHOSIS

Information to candidates:

Name of patient: Mrs Heiner

Mrs Heiner has been arrested by the police officers following her confrontation with her neighbours and currently being sent to the emergency department for further medical and psychiatric assessment. You are the core trainee-3 on call, and you are tasked to speak to her to determine if she has any psychiatric conditions that might necessitate invoking the appropriate sections to keep her in the hospital.

Task: Please speak to Mrs Heiner and perform a mental state examination.

Outline of station:

You are Mrs Heiner, and you are frustrated as to why you're the one in the hospital and not your neighbours. Your neighbours have been troubling you for the past year or so, ever since they moved into the apartment near yours. You frequently hear them speaking about you and often make demeaning remarks about you. You know that they are doing so because they want to get rid of you, to occupy your apartment. You hear them most clearly at the wall separating your apartment from theirs. You believe that the food you cook in the house tastes strange as you firmly believe that your neighbours have poisoned the food you cook. You are only able to eat out.

You have previously complained to the police, but they took no action. You approached your local district council, but the officer did not believe you. You have been feeling increasingly troubled, and you have decided that you need to do something about this issue. You have decided to confront them today. You have used your walking stick to threaten them not to bother you further. At the start of the interview, you should be frustrated that you have been arrested and not your neighbours. You do not wish to speak to a psychiatrist as you firmly believe you do not have any mental health condition.

CASC Construct Table:

The CASC Construct Table is formatted such that candidates would be able adequately to cover both the range and depth of the assessment required in this station.

DOI: 10.1201/9781003313113-40

Approach: Be prepared for a patient who might be frustrated and unwilling to share more information. Demonstration of empathy is crucial towards eliciting the symptomatology. Starting off: "Hello, I am Dr Melvyn, one of the psychiatrists from the mental health unit. I understand that the police have brought you in today. Could we have a chat about this?"			
Clarification of history of presenting complaint	It does sound like you have been having a challenging time. Can you tell me more so that I can better understand your situation?	I'm sorry to learn about the difficult circumstances that you have been through.	Could you tell me how long you feel your neighbours have been troubling you? Have you sought any form of help?
Exploring auditory hallucinations/ exploring delusional beliefs	Could you tell me more about the voices that you have been hearing? Are they as clear as our current conversation? What do they say?	Do they speak directly to you? Can you give me examples of what they have been saying to you?	Do they refer to you as he or she, or do they call you by your name? Do they comment on what you are doing? Do they give you commands as to what to do? Could any alternative explanations help account for these experiences that you have been having?
Eliciting hallucinations in all other modalities	Have you noticed that the food or the drink seemed to have a different taste recently? Has there been anything wrong with your sense of smell?	Have you had any strange experiences or feelings in your body recently?	Have you been able to see things that other people cannot see? What kind of things could you see? Could you give me an example?
Elicit thought disorders	Do you feel that your thoughts are being interfered with? Who do you think is doing all this?	Do you have thoughts in your head that you feel are not your own thoughts? Where do you think these thoughts come from?	Do you feel that your thoughts are being broadcasted such that others would know what you are thinking? Do you feel that some external forces take your thoughts away from your head?
Elicit passivity experiences	Do you feel in control of your own actions and emotions?	Do you feel that someone or something is trying to control you?	Who do you think this would be?

(Continued)

(Continued)

Impact of symptoms on mood and coping mechanisms	It has been a difficult time for you. How have you been coping? How has your memory been? Any visual or auditory impairment?	How has this affected your mood? Are you still interested in things that you used to enjoy? Are there any difficulties with your sleep or appetite?	Have you made use of any substance, such as alcohol, to help you to cope? What about street drugs?
Risk assessment	Could you tell me more as to why the police have been involved today?	Do you currently still have any plans or thoughts to confront your neighbours?	Are you so stressed with all these experiences that you might think of ending it all?

Common pitfalls:

a. Failure to be empathetic enough to engage the frustrated patient.
b. Failure to cover the range and depth of the task—need to demonstrate to the college examiner that you have explored all the other modalities of hallucinations and tried to elicit the rest of the first-rank symptoms.

Information to candidates:

Name of patient: Mrs Heiner

Mrs Heiner has been assessed by the medical team and deemed to be medically well. She has been seen by the consultant psychiatrist and deemed to have late-onset psychosis. She has been commenced on an antipsychotic called olanzapine 5 mg at night. Her brother, Mr Smith, has called in requesting to speak to the team as he has some concerns about his sister's condition. He is keen to understand how the team intends to manage his sister's condition.

Task: Please speak to Mr Smith and address all his concerns and expectations.

Outline of station:

You are Mr Smith, the brother of Mrs Heiner. Your sister was widowed two years ago, and you are her only relative. You have previously heard about her being arrested by the police, and you have heard that, following the arrest, she was transferred to a hospital and currently being sectioned for treatment. You are keen to know more about her diagnosis and the potential causes for her current condition. You understand that your sister has been commenced on medication, but you are also wondering whether there are other alternatives apart from medication. You want to know more about the medication (olanzapine), and you also wish to know more about the longer-term treatment. You wish to know if she needs alternative housing or placement.

CASC Construct Table:

The CASC Construct Table is formatted such that candidates would be able adequately to cover both the range and depth of the assessment required in this station.

DOI: 10.1201/9781003313113-41

Starting off: "Hello, I am Dr Melvyn, one of the psychiatrists from the mental health unit. I understand that you have some concerns about your sister's condition. Could we have a chat?"		
Clarification about diagnosis	I understand that it must be a difficult time for you. I'm here to explain and to clarify any doubts that you have.	With the symptoms that your sister has shared with us, it seems like what she has is late-onset psychosis. Have you heard about it before?	Late-onset psychosis is the same as schizophrenia. Schizophrenia is a common mental health disorder affecting how one thinks, feels, and behaves.
Explain aetiology	There are many causes for this condition. It is tough to identify the exact cause of your sister's condition.	If there is a known family history of schizophrenia, your sister might be predisposed to it.	Often, those with paranoid personality disorders as well as hearing impairments might be predisposed as well. Does she have any visual impairment as well?
Explain treatment options	You're right to mention that there are both inpatient and outpatient treatment options.	To determine which is more suitable, we need to perform an assessment of risks. In your sister's case, there is an element of risk as she has confronted her neighbours.	As your sister did not have had much insight into her condition, there is thus a need for the team to detain her under the Mental Health Act.
Explain pharmacological treatment	I'm sure you're aware that your sister has been started on a medication known as olanzapine. Have you heard about it before?	Olanzapine is a commonly used antipsychotic medication. It works for patients with late-onset psychosis by regulating the amount of brain chemicals such as dopamine in the brain.	Like all medication, antipsychotics do have their own side effects. The common side effects include sedation and weight gain. We usually would recommend a continuation of the medication for at least six months.
Explain alternative treatments	Apart from medication, the other alternative form of treatment would be that of psychological or talking therapies. Have you heard of that before?	Cognitive behavioural therapy could be helpful for your sister when she is more settled, as she would be able to learn techniques to cope with her symptoms.	If sensory impairments are a concern, we could refer your sister to our specialist colleagues to help her with her impairments.
Explain long-term management	In the long term, we hope that we can get your sister our multidisciplinary team involvement.	We hope that our community psychiatric nurse can help support her and watch her medication adherence in the community.	If you do have concerns about her current accommodation, we could also consider alternatives, such as shelter housing. Alternatively, we might recommend your sister attend day centres to keep her engaged.

Common pitfalls:

a. Failure to explain the rationale as to why the patient needs compulsory treatment.
b. Failure to explain other non-pharmacological management, such as looking into and helping the patient with her sensory impairments.
c. Failure to cover and explain the long-term management of the patient.

Information to candidates:

Name of patient: Mr Johns

Mr Johns has been a resident in the nursing home for the previous six months. Recently, over the past week or so, the nursing staff have noted that Mr Johns has been increasing agitated during the day. There was an episode to which Mr Johns attempted to hit one of the staff and another nursing home resident. The support worker has been informed about his changes in behaviour.

Task: Please speak to Mr Johns' support worker to obtain more collateral information to arrive at a possible diagnosis.

Outline of station:

You are Sarah, the support worker of Mr Johns. You have known him since the day he was transferred to your nursing home. Over the past one week or so, you have heard from the staff that he has increasingly difficult behaviours. You have not identified any specific triggers prior to the episodes of aggression. You know that Mr Johns has a history of Alzheimer's dementia, and he was last seen by the old age psychiatrist around three months ago. Per the memo from the specialist, there was no worsening in his symptoms or functioning, and the specialist also does not feel that there are any associated comorbid psychiatric disorders. You know that Mr Johns has not been sick recently. You understand from the staff that there have been two new residents in the nursing home over the past week. In addition, due to Mr Johns' wife being sick, she has not visited him for the past two weeks. You are keen to share as much information as possible with the doctor as you hope that Mr Johns' condition could improve, or else it would be tough for the nursing home to continue having him.

CASC Construct Table:

The CASC Construct Table is formatted such that candidates would be able adequately to cover both the range and depth of the assessment required in this station.

DOI: 10.1201/9781003313113-42

Starting off: "Hello, I am Dr Melvyn, one of the psychiatrists from the mental health unit. I understand that you have some concerns about Mr Johns, one of your residents in your home, due to changes in his behaviours. Could we have a chat about this?"			
Clarification of behavioural changes	I understand that it has been difficult for you and your nursing staff. Could you please tell me more about the difficulties? How long have you noticed these changes to be?	Have you noticed any changes in his mood? You mentioned that there are times to when he seemed more irritable. Are there specific triggers?	Has he been verbally or physically violent towards your staff or other residents? Could you tell me more? Are his behaviours progressively getting worse?
Exploration of psychiatric symptoms	Could you share with me the reasons why he needed placement in your nursing home? What was the diagnosis that was given to Mr Johnson previously?	Has he been regular with his follow-up appointments with the psychiatrist? Has the psychiatrist started him or changed any of his medication? What did the psychiatrist say about his condition during the latest follow-up appointment?	Does he appear to be more emotional than usual? Is he still able to enjoy things that he used to enjoy? Are there times when your staff have noticed him responding to things or talking to himself? Has he been keeping to himself and not interacting with others?
Exploration of physical symptoms	Has he been unwell recently? Does he have any pre-existing medical conditions? Does he have any hearing or vision impairment?	Did he spike a temperature in the past week or so? Did he have any recent falls?	Is he in any form of pain? Is he able to clear his bowels and pass urine without any issues?
Exploration of environmental changes	Have there been any changes in your nursing home?	Is there new staff in your nursing home? Or are there new staff attending to his needs?	Have there been any changes to the regular routine in the nursing home? Have there been any changes in the structured activities usually conducted in the home?
Exploration of social changes/ lack of visitors	How does he usually spend his time in the nursing home?	Has his family visited him recently?	

Common pitfalls:

a. This might seem to be an easy station as, basically, candidates only need to elicit information from the support worker. However, candidates need to have a structure as to what information they need to gather from the support worker.

b. Candidates need to cover the range and depth of the task adequately—they need to explore the psychiatric symptoms, rule out physical problems, and assess environmental changes and social environment changes. They also need to check whether there have been changes in the structured activities in the home.

Information to candidates:

Name of patient: Mr Johns

Mr Johns has been a resident in the nursing home for the previous six months. Over the past week or so, the nursing staff have noted that Mr Johns has been increasingly agitated during the day. There was an episode in which Mr Johns attempted to hit one of the staff and another nursing home resident. The support worker has been informed about his changes in behaviour. You have obtained further information from the support worker in the previous station. Mr Johns' son now demands to speak to you. He is distraught that the team has started his father on an antipsychotic medication known as olanzapine. He wishes to know more about the management plans that the team has for his father.

Task: Please speak to Mr Johns' son and address all his concerns and expectations.

Outline of station:

You are Tom, Mr Johns' son. You have heard about the issues in the nursing home. You understand that the team has decided to start your father on a medication known as olanzapine. You have read up on the medication on the Internet, and it seems to be a very dangerous medication for use in the elderly. You are frustrated that the team went ahead and started the medication without informing you. You are very concerned about the increased risk of stroke that the medication has. You wonder how long the team would be continuing the medication. You are not very keen for your father to be on medication. You expect the core trainee to discuss with you other options apart from medication.

CASC Construct Table:

The CASC Construct Table is formatted such that candidates would be able adequately to cover both the range and depth of the assessment required in this station.

DOI: 10.1201/9781003313113-43

Starting off: "Hello, I am Dr Melvyn, one of the psychiatrists from the mental health unit. I understand that you have some concerns about your father, Mr Johns. I am hoping we can have a chat about this."			
Clarification of chief concerns	I apologize. The team should have kept you informed that your father has been commenced on antipsychotic medication.	I hear that you have some concerns about the medication—olanzapine. Could you tell me more?	(Or) Could you share with me your understanding of olanzapine?
Explain the rationale for the commencement of antipsychotics	I understand that you're deeply concerned about your father's condition. Could I tell you more as to why the team has come to such a decision?	As you know, your dad has Alzheimer's dementia, and this is a condition that affects one's cognitive functioning as well as his behaviours. In Alzheimer's dementia, there is a deterioration in one's cognition and daily functioning gradually. This is at times accompanied by behavioural changes, such as aggression and agitation. At times, individuals might also present with delusions of theft, sleep disturbances, any other inappropriate sexual behaviours, and wandering.	I hope you understand that there was a situation last week to which your father's and others' safety were compromised. Despite the staff's efforts to calm him down, he was still quite agitated and aggressive, and hence, the team needed to start him on olanzapine to calm him down.
Clarification of side effects of antipsychotics and duration of use	I understand that you are very concerned about side effects of the medication. Like all medication, olanzapine does also have its side effects.	It is true that the medication does predispose your father to an increased chance of strokes. In addition, the other common side effects of the medication include that of sedation and weight gain.	Prior to the commencement of any medication, the team usually weighs the risks/benefits ratio before starting. In your father's case, the benefits clearly outweigh the risks of him injuring himself. We have started him on the lowest possible dose of medication and will monitor him closely for side effects. The team is not planning to continue the medication on a long-term basis. Once your father has calmed down and responded to other interventions, the team would consider discontinuing the treatment.

| Explain non-pharmacological options | Apart from the usage of medication, the team is hoping that other forms of treatments may be useful for your father. These include reality orientation—which involves the consistent usage of orientation devices to remind patients of their environment. | Reminiscent therapy involves reliving past experiences using old television sets and radios. Art therapy, aromatherapy, and music therapy might be helpful as well. | We will speak to our multidisciplinary team and try to organize a schedule of activities for your father to keep him consistently engaged. We recommend that your mother visit him regularly as it would also be helpful for him. In the meantime, we would ensure that we have more staff and that he has more supervision from the staff. Do you have any questions for me? |

Common pitfalls:

a. Failure to engage with an angry relative by demonstrating adequate empathy and understanding of his concerns.

b. Failure to explain clearly why the team has decided for commencement of antipsychotic medication (need to mention the specific risks and that the team has considered the risk/benefits ratio).

c. Failure to explain alternatives to pharmacological treatment.

Information to candidates:

Name of patient: Mr Mitchell

Mr Mitchell is a 75-year-old gentleman recently diagnosed with Alzheimer's dementia. He has been started on anti-dementia medication to help slow down the progression of his symptoms. Brian, his son, has accompanied him today for his routine follow-up. Brian is turning 50 years old this year and is very concerned that his father has been diagnosed with Alzheimer's dementia. He is worried about acquiring the illness himself. He would like to clarify his concerns with a doctor.

Task: Please speak to Mr Mitchell's son and address all his concerns and expectations.

Outline of station:

You are Brian, the son of Mr Mitchell. You understand from the doctor recently that your father has been diagnosed with Alzheimer's dementia. You are very concerned about him being given this diagnosis. You wonder what the difference between Alzheimer's dementia and dementia is. You would like to know more about how your father would progress as the conditions worsen. In addition, you are very worried about you acquiring the same disorder. You want to hear more about the genetic risk of acquiring the disorder from the doctor. In addition, you want to know all the causes of the disorder. If there is an underlying genetic linkage, you wish to ask if blood and genetic testing would help. You want to check with the doctor whether other specific lifestyle changes, such as eating a special diet, would reduce your risks.

CASC Construct Table:

The CASC Construct Table is formatted such that candidates would be able adequately to cover both the range and depth of the assessment required in this station.

DOI: 10.1201/9781003313113-44

Starting off: "Hello, I am Dr Melvyn, one of the psychiatrists from the mental health unit. I understand that you have some concerns about your father, Mr Mitchell. I am hoping we could have a chat about this."			
Clarifications about the diagnosis of the patient	I'm sorry to be informing you that your father has been diagnosed with Alzheimer's dementia. We have since started him on some medication to help with slowing down the progression of memory loss.	Have you heard about Alzheimer's dementia before? Alzheimer's dementia is the commonest type of dementia. However, the terminology "dementia," is a general term and there are various types of dementia. In essence, dementia refers to a condition that usually starts off with memory difficulties. In time to come, it might get worse as other areas of the brain are involved. As a result, there might be impairments and difficulties with coping with daily tasks.	Whilst medication could help him with his symptoms, other non-medication approaches include environmental modification and behavioural interventions. Environmental modification could include reducing distractions, adjusting ambient temperatures, and improving access to toilets. In behavioural interventions, individuals are encouraged to participate in activities that they previously find to be enjoyable and meaningful.
Address the main concern about risk	I understand that you are concerned about your chances of acquiring the same disorder.	The risk would be approximately three to four times higher for children whose parents have dementia.	It's hard to predict whether you will acquire dementia. In a small minority of individuals, dementia appears to be transmitted from generation to generation. However, this is rare and accounts for 1% of all cases of Alzheimer's dementia.
Address concerns about blood and genetic testing	Apo-lipoprotein E has been discovered to be responsible for one's susceptibility towards getting the disorder.	I understand that you are concerned about whether there are blood tests or genetic tests that could tell whether there's a chance you would get the disorder.	Unfortunately, the current blood test and genetic testing are not diagnostic and have a limited role in predicting whether you would acquire the same disorder.
Clarifications about other factors that would predispose to Alzheimer's dementia	The chances of one having Alzheimer's dementia increase as one gets older.	Individuals with a previous history of head injury, previous episodes of depression and lower education are more susceptible towards acquiring dementia.	In addition, individuals with Down's syndrome are more susceptible towards acquiring Alzheimer's dementia.

(Continued)

(Continued)

Address any other concerns	There has not been much evidence regarding smoking and how it might protect against Alzheimer's dementia.	Also, there is no concrete evidence about special diets and their protective effect against dementia.	

Common pitfalls:

a. Failure to explain Alzheimer's dementia in a non-technical way.
b. Failure to briefly mention non-pharmacological options for the management of behavioural disturbances.
c. Failure to explore all the concerns of the relative.
d. Failure to state specifically the exact increment in risk of acquiring dementia.

STATION 45
HISTORY
TAKING—DEMENTIA

Information to candidates:

Name of patient: Mr Casey

Mr Casey has been referred to your service by his local GP as he has been having problems with his memory over the past year or so. He is here today with his wife, Sandra.

Task: Please speak to his wife, Sandra, and obtain a history to arrive at a possible diagnosis.

Outline of station:

You are Sandra, the wife of Mr Casey. You have noticed that your husband has been having increasing memory difficulties over the past year. It has progressively worsened over the past two months, and you are increasingly concerned as you are the only caregiver staying with him. He seemed to have a lot of trouble with his short-term memory. He muddles up dates and times. He has difficulties at times recognizing your grandchildren as well. In addition, you have noticed that, over the past two months, he has been having difficulties with finding the right words during some conversations. He is still able to dress and groom himself. You are concerned that, over the past two months, he is increasingly forgetful, and that has led to some issues. For example, he has once forgotten his way back home after his early morning walk. In addition, there was an occasion in which he forgot to turn off the kettle as he could not remember that he had boiled some water. Thus far, there have not been other behavioural issues, such as any aggression or self-harm episodes.

CASC Construct Table:

The CASC Construct Table is formatted such that candidates would be able adequately to cover both the range and depth of the assessment required in this station.

DOI: 10.1201/9781003313113-45

Starting off: "Hello, I am Dr Melvyn, one of the psychiatrists from the mental health unit. I understand that you have some concerns about your husband. I am hoping we can have a chat about this."			
Clarification about presenting complaint	I understand that the GP has referred your husband over as there have been some concerns about his memory difficulties. Could you please tell me more?	Could you tell me when these memory difficulties first started? (Or) How long have there been difficulties with his memory?	How have things been recently? I'm sorry to hear that it has been getting worse. It must have been a very difficult time for you.
Exploration of memory difficulties	Have there been any problems with his short-term memory? By that, I mean, are there times to which he misplaces things? Have there been times to which he forgets his meals? Has he ever tried to hide or cover up his memory problem by providing a made-up answer?	What about his memories of things in the past? Could he still remember things that happened years ago?	Onset and progression— gradual or sudden? Any previous head injury? Any medical problems (e.g. high blood pressure, high cholesterol, stroke/ transient ischaemic attacks)? Any low mood prior to memory problems (pseudodementia)?
Exploration of orientation and visuospatial dysfunction	Does he seem to get muddled up with the day and dates?	Have there been times to when you noticed that he seemed very confused?	Is he able to recognize his loved ones? What about distant relatives that he hardly meets?
Exploration of language, communication, and recognition difficulties	Have there been times to when he has difficulties finding the right words in a conversation?	Are there times when he seemed to have great difficulties understanding a normal conversation?	Is he able to recognize and identify everyday objects? Can he find the right words to name those objects?
Exploration of functioning	Is he still able to manage himself? Could you tell me more about the difficulties that he has been having?	Does he need additional help with any of the following? – Dressing – Washing – Toileting – Ambulation	Does he need additional help with any of the following? – Finances – Shopping – Food preparation – Transportation

Risk assessment	Have there been any other concerns with regard to his behaviour of late?	Has he wandered out of the house previously? Has he ever got lost when he was out of the house? Any fire/flooding accidents (from failing to turn off stove/taps)? Any financial exploitation by others? Any abuse from caregivers?	Has he been aggressive verbally or physically at home? Has he accidentally hurt himself recently?

Common pitfalls:

a. Failure to demonstrate empathy when the caregiver shares the history and the account of the difficulties she has been experiencing.

b. Failure to cover the range and the depth of the task.

**It would be worthwhile to distinguish whether the symptoms are due to AD or a vascular nature.

The following is an example of a CASC station that requires the candidate to extract more information to come to a diagnosis of vascular dementia:

Name of patient: Mr Stevens

His GP has referred Mr Stevens to the specialist memory clinic. His son, Joseph, reports that his father has been having difficulties with his memory for the past one year.

Task: Please speak to his son, Joseph, and obtain as much history as possible to arrive at a diagnosis.

Outline of station:

You are Joseph, the son of Mr Stevens. You have noticed that over the past year, your father's memory has been declining. He has been having problems with the immediate recall of information, especially so with his short-term memory. He cannot recognize your distant relatives at times. Otherwise, he is still able to care for himself, but perhaps not as well as before as it seems that he needs more assistance from your mother. You know that he has a long-standing history of poorly controlled blood pressure and diabetes mellitus. He had a minor cerebrovascular event around two years ago, to which his neurologist has recommended that he has to be maintained on lifelong warfarin treatment.

Please consider the following additional questions to help distinguish AD with that of vascular dementia:

Clarify medical history	Does your father have any chronic medical conditions that I need to know of?	Thanks for sharing with me. Could I know more about the control of his medical conditions? Did his doctor tell you what his medical conditions were?	Has he had stroke before? Have there been scans done previously? How has he been since the onset of his stroke? Has his stroke led to any functional impairments?

Common pitfalls:

a. Failure to ask for adequate information to cover the range and the depth of the station.
b. Failure to ask for the previous history of medical conditions.
c. Failure to ask for residual impairments after the onset of his previous cerebrovascular accident.

STATION 46
ANTI-DEMENTIA DRUGS

Information to candidates:

Name of patient: Mr Podgorski

Mr Podgorski has been recently referred by his GP to the old age psychiatry service as he has been having increasing difficulties with his memory over the past year. The old age consultant has decided to start Mr Podgorski on one anti-dementia drug, donepezil. His son, Jonathan, is here today and wants to discuss the medication he started. Jonathan has read up about the medication on the Internet and is concerned about the side effects of the medication.

Task: Please speak to his son, Jonathan, and address all his concerns and expectations.

Outline of station:

You are Jonathan, the son of Mr Podgorski. Your father has been diagnosed with Alzheimer's dementia recently, and he has since been started on an anti-dementia medication known as donepezil. You have read up about the medication on the Internet, and you are concerned about the side effects associated with the medication. You wish to know the duration of treatment and the effectiveness of this medication for patients. You wish to know more about the outpatient follow-up as well as the investigations that are required during each visit. You are concerned about the effects the medication might have on the liver, and you are also concerned about the cost of the medication. You have read from the internet that psychiatric medication is addictive, and you do not want your father to be on any addictive medication.

CASC Construct Table:

The CASC Construct Table is formatted such that candidates would be able adequately to cover both the range and depth of the assessment required in this station.

DOI: 10.1201/9781003313113-46

Starting off: "Hello, I am Dr Melvyn, one of the psychiatrists from the mental health unit. I understand that you have some concerns about your father. I am hoping we can have a chat about this."			
Clarification about anti-dementia drugs	I understand that you have some concerns about the medication that we have started your father on. The medication we have started is called donepezil. It is one of the anti-dementia drugs. Have you heard about it before?	Thanks for sharing your understanding and your concerns about the medication with me. Unfortunately, anti-dementia drugs would not cure your father of his dementia.	However, it could help to slow down the progression of his current condition. It could help him with his mood, motivation, and his alertness.
Explain the duration of treatment and efficacy	Anti-dementia drugs work on chemicals in the brain. When an individual has dementia, there is a reduction in the amount of a particular brain chemical known as acetylcholine.	Anti-dementia drugs help to increase the levels of this chemical. It is thus hoped that by increasing the levels of this chemical, it would help to stabilize the memory and the functioning of your father.	Previous research has shown that approximately 40–50% of individuals do respond to the medication. We will regularly monitor your father's cognition and memory using a memory test and decide whether he would benefit from the drug.
Explain the side effects of donepezil	Like any other medication, anti-dementia drugs also have their side effects. Before starting the medication, we need to consider the patient's medical history. Donepezil is contraindicated for patients with asthma.	The most common side effects include that of feelings of nausea, diarrhoea, and urinary incontinence. Some patients might complain of insomnia and muscle cramps. Other side effects might include the risk of slowing down the heart rate.	
Clarify the follow-up required and investigations needed	We will usually start patients on the lowest dose of the medication and aim to get them early in our outpatient clinic to see whether they can tolerate the medication.	If they are tolerating well, we might gradually increase the dosage. We would aim to see your father every six months.	During the subsequent visitations, we will perform a memory test known as the mini-mental state examination (MMSE). This test helps us understand the extent of cognitive deficits. We will continue the medication if the test scores are more than 10/30.

| Address concerns | Do you have any other concerns regarding the medication in general or donepezil in particular? I do wish to inform you that the NHS covers the costs of the medication. | Thanks for highlighting your concerns. Anti-dementia medication is not addictive. They usually do not affect liver functioning. If he cannot tolerate donepezil, we could consider another class of anti-dementia medications, memantine. This medication works on other chemicals in the brain. | The advantage of donepezil is that the frequency of administration is once per day. If your father does not wish to take the tablets, we might need to consider alternative medication available in the form of patches. I know that we have discussed quite a lot today. I would like to offer you some leaflets. |

Common pitfalls:

a. Failure to determine and establish the baseline understanding that the caregiver might have.

b. Failure to cover the range and the depth of the task.

Information to candidates:

Name of patient: Mr Northey

Mr Northey is a 75-year-old retired teacher who was diagnosed with Parkinson's disease six months ago. In addition to the symptoms of Parkinson's disease that he is suffering from, his family members have noted that his memory has declined over the past few months. A recent DaTSCAN was done, which showed features consistent with that of Lewy body dementia.

Task: Please speak to his daughter, Sally, to clarify the diagnosis and to explain the treatment options for this condition.

Outline of station:

You are Sally, the daughter of Mr Northey. You do not live together with your father, but you are aware that he was diagnosed with Parkinson's disease six months ago following a fall at home. He has multiple features of Parkinson's disease. However, you have noticed that his memory has not been as good as previously. He cannot remember your girl's name, despite her frequently visiting. Your mother has mentioned that he is especially bad with the recall of immediate events and things discussed. At times, your mother has noticed that he has been responding to visual hallucinations. This has been a cause of concern for all. You want to know the exact diagnosis that your father has. You have queries as to whether the doctors might have misdiagnosed, and this might just be Parkinson's disease–related dementia (based on your own research, you have found out that individuals with Parkinson's disease do have dementia as well). You are curious as to what will be the best choice regarding medication for your father. You are especially concerned about falls, and you will share this only if the candidate remembers to ask for your other concerns and expectations.

CASC Construct Table:

The CASC Construct Table is formatted such that candidates would be able adequately to cover both the range and depth of the assessment required in this station.

DOI: 10.1201/9781003313113-47

Starting off: "Hello, I am Dr Melvyn, one of the psychiatrists from the mental health unit. I understand that you have some concerns about your father. I am hoping we can have a chat about this."			
Clarification of diagnosis	I understand that it must have been a challenging time for you and your family.	Based on the specialized scan results, your father has a form of dementia known as Lewy body dementia.	Have you heard about this form of dementia before? It is the third most common cause of late-onset dementia and commonly affects more men than women.
Explain common clinical manifestations	This form of dementia has three classical symptoms, which include that of falls, fluctuating scores in memory testing (fluctuating cognition), and visual hallucinations.	With regards to cognition, individuals with the disorder tend to have fluctuating cognition, and short-term memory is less affected in the early stages. The common noncognitive features include that of depression, hallucinations (usually complex visual hallucinations), and delusions.	There might be other associated changes, such as progressive loss of facial expression, changes in strength and tone of the voice, slowness, muscle stiffness, trembling of the limbs, and a tendency to shuffle when walking.
Explain possible aetiological causes	The exact cause is still uncertain.	The memory impairments and the changes are likely to be due to the presence of Lewy bodies in the brain.	It is believed that the presence of these deposits would influence the action of some of the important chemicals in the brain.
Clarification of the differences with Parkinson's disease dementia	Thanks for sharing with me your understanding of Parkinson's disease and its associated memory problems.	Based on the clinical history and the brain scan results, our team is not inclined to think this is Parkinson's disease dementia.	For Parkinson's disease–related dementia, the cognitive symptoms tend to occur at least one year after developing extrapyramidal signs.
Explain management options	Antipsychotics are usually not used due to the risk of severe adverse reactions.	Anti-dementia medication is usually considered for patients with significant noncognitive symptoms that have led to significant distress or challenging behaviours. Rivastigmine has the best-researched evidence to date and could help with the cognitive symptoms, the delusions, and hallucinations.	Anti-parkinsonism medication could be used to help with motor symptoms. We like to work closely with the neurologist to adjust the medication doses accordingly.

(Continued)

(Continued)

Address concerns	I know that I have shared a lot today. Do you have any questions for me?	I hear your concerns about the risk of falls for your father.	I would like to recommend that he be referred to our multidisciplinary team. The occupational therapist could help to look into environmental modifications to reduce the risk associated with falls.

Common pitfalls:

a. Failure to explain in depth with regards to the clinical manifestation of LBD.
b. Failure to clearly clarify the differences between Parkinson's disease–related dementia with that of Lewy body dementia.
c. Failure to elicit other concerns and address them accordingly.

Information to candidates:

Name of patient: Mr Northey

Mr Northey is a 75-year-old retired teacher diagnosed with Parkinson's disease six months ago. In addition to the symptoms of Parkinson's disease that he is suffering from, his family members have noted that his memory has declined over the past few months. A recent DaTSCAN was carried out, which showed features consistent with that of Lewy body dementia. His daughter, Sally, has been told of his diagnosis previously. Her husband, Bobby, is here today and hopes to see the doctor urgently as he needs help with managing his father-in-law. Mr Northey has been started on rivastigmine 3 mg daily previously and was better. However, in the past couple of weeks, his condition has deteriorated. He is noted to be increasingly confused and responding to visual hallucinations.

Task: Please speak to his son-in-law, Bobby, and address all his concerns and expectations.

Outline of station:

You are Bobby, the son-in-law of Mr Northey. You learnt more about his diagnosis from your wife around one year ago. You know that your father-in-law has been started on medication that was helpful for his symptoms previously. However, in the past few weeks or so, you have noticed that his condition has drastically changed for the worst. He is increasingly confused and would have a sleep-wake reversal. At times, in the middle of the night, he would become very agitated whilst responding to visual hallucinations. Sally, your wife, is out of town, and you are the only caregiver for the next couple of weeks. You want to know what you could do to help your father-in-law with his condition. You wish to know the possible reasons for his current condition. In addition, you are hoping that the doctor could adjust or start him on new medication, such as antipsychotics, to help him with his condition. You also wish to know what else could be beneficial for him. You desperately need answers and hope that the candidate can understand the difficulties you are facing.

CASC Construct Table:

The CASC Construct Table is formatted such that candidates would be able adequately to cover both the range and depth of the assessment required in this station.

DOI: 10.1201/9781003313113-48

*It is also the objective of this station to highlight the variations in clinical management among individuals presenting with varying subtypes of dementia.

Starting off: "Hello, I am Dr Melvyn, one of the psychiatrists from the mental health unit. I understand that you have some concerns about your father-in-law. I am hoping we can have a chat about this."			
Establishing rapport	I'm sorry to learn about what has been happening. It must be a challenging time for you.	I'm hoping that we can do our best to help you with the care needs of your father-in-law.	Do you think you will be willing to undergo a carer assessment? (Or) We'd like to discuss your father-in-law's case with the rest of the members of our multidisciplinary team. Our community psychiatric nurse could help by visiting your home and offering some interventions. How does that sound for you?
Establish likely causes for changes in behaviour	Could you tell me more about how he has been? How long have you noticed these changes? Are these behaviours new in nature, or have you noticed them before? Sometimes when there is a progression of underlying dementia, there might be worsening of these symptoms.	Has the neurologist seen him recently? Have there been any recent adjustments in his Parkinson's medication?	Has he been taken ill recently? Have any changes or decline in his physical functioning and health recently?
Discuss pharmacological treatment options	At times adjustment of medication might help with his behavioural difficulties. For example, did he previously respond well to the anti-dementia medication? We could consider increasing the dose of the anti-dementia medication to help him with his current condition.	If there has been a recent change in his Parkinsonism medication by his neurologist, it might be worthwhile for an early review by his neurologist. Sometimes adjustment of the medication could result in behavioural changes as well.	I understand that you feel a sleeping medication might help him with his behaviour. However, we would not recommend it, given that there is a high risk of falls associated with the usage of the medication. In addition, regular usage might lead to dependency.

(Variations in management for the other subtypes of dementia)	Vascular dementia The local NICE guidelines do not recommend using any anti-dementia medication for vascular dementia. It is advised that we help him gain better control of his underlying medical condition (for example, better control of his blood pressure, cholesterol problems, and diabetes). The local GP who is following up on your father's condition could help by prescribing appropriate medication to help optimize his condition.	Frontotemporal dementia There is no specific pharmacological intervention for cognitive impairments in this form of dementia. Selective serotonin reuptake inhibitors (SSRIs) or other antidepressants are indicated for non-cognitive features.	
Discuss non-pharmacological treatment options	Apart from medication, other techniques might be beneficial and helpful to deal with the current behavioural difficulties that you are facing.	Such techniques might include the usage of aromatherapy as well as regular re-orientation.	Vascular dementia Apart from medication, we hope we can slow down the progression by encouraging your father to modify his lifestyle. We'd like to recommend that he participate in regular exercises, as well as cut down on smoking or drinking (if he is doing so).
Address all other concerns	We have spoken a lot today. Do you have any questions for me?	I think your concern about the usage of an antipsychotic is valid. Usually, we would not consider using an antipsychotic in view of the adverse effects associated with its use.	However, if the behaviours are indeed severe and distressing and all other measures have failed, we might consider a very low dose of quetiapine. However, we need to watch carefully for side effects as patients with LBD are prone to side effects as they are more sensitive to these neuroleptics.

Common pitfalls:

a. Failure to empathize and discuss the relative alternatives management plans to help him with the care arrangement of his father-in-law.

b. Failure to consider other causes for the acute changes in behaviour (hence failing to cover the range and the depth needed for the station adequately).

c. Failure to consider titration of the dose of the parkinsonism medication (as changes in the dose of the medication might cause behavioural changes).

d. Failure to consider and explain non-pharmacological alternatives.

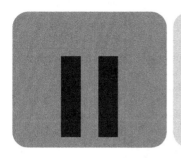

Information to candidates:

Name of patient: Mr Meyer

Mr Meyer, a 60-year-old man, has been referred by his GP to the old age psychiatry service. His family has noticed that he has had personality changes over the last two years. He has been increasingly socially disinhibited and would at times have sexually inappropriate behaviours. These behavioural changes are in addition to there being a progressive worsening of his memory. He is also having difficulties with planning his daily routine. His wife, the main caregiver, is extremely distressed by his condition and wants some help from your service.

Task: Please speak to his wife, Mrs Sally Meyer, and take a history to come to an eventual diagnosis.

Outline of station:

You are Sally, the wife of Mr Meyer. Over the past year, you have noticed that your husband's memory has been failing. On several occasions, he seemed unable to recall conversations you just have had with him. In addition, there have been occasions to which he has sexually inappropriate behaviours. On one occasion, you were attending a church service with him, and he openly made inappropriate sexual remarks to another female who was in the same service. In addition, you have noticed that he has difficulties recognizing your distant relatives. He has word-finding difficulties as well. He does seem to need more help with his daily activities. There was another occasion to which he wandered out of the house and could not find his way back. You are very worried about his condition and wonder how best you could help him. You are very distressed and would share more only if the candidate is empathetic towards you.

CASC Construct Table:

The CASC Construct Table is formatted such that candidates would be able adequately to cover both the range and depth of the assessment required in this station.

Starting off: "Hello, I am Dr Melvyn, one of the psychiatrists from the mental health unit. I understand that you have some concerns about your husband. I am hoping we could have a chat about this."			
Clarification about presenting complaint	I understand that the GP has referred your husband as there have been some concerns about his memory difficulties and the changes in his behaviours. Could you please tell me more?	Could you tell me when these memory and behavioural difficulties first started? (Or) How long have there been difficulties with his memory?	How have things been recently? I'm sorry to hear that it has been getting worse. It must have been a very difficult time for you.
Exploration of frontal lobe symptoms	I am sorry to hear how distressing it has been for you. Can you describe to me how your husband has been in terms of his personality previously? How has that changed?	Is he able to plan what he wants to do for the day? Has he been more impulsive recently? Does he seem to keep repeating particular words or actions? Is he able to recognize familiar faces? Does he have any problems recognizing objects? Is he able to shift from task to task easily?	Has he done anything embarrassing? Or anything that is sexually inappropriate? Can you tell me more?
Exploration of memory difficulties	Have there been any problems with his short-term memory? By that, I mean, are there times to which he misplaces things? Have there been times to which he forgets his meals?	What about his memories of things in the past? Could he still remember things that happened years ago?	
Exploration of orientation and visuospatial dysfunction	Does he seem to get muddled up with the day and dates?	Have there been times when you noticed that he seemed very confused?	Is he able to recognize his loved ones? What about distant relatives that he hardly meets?
Exploration of language, communication, and recognition difficulties	Have there been times when he has difficulties finding the right words in a conversation?	Are there times when he seemed to have great difficulties understanding a normal conversation?	Is he able to recognize and identify everyday objects? Can he find the right words to name those objects?

Exploration of functioning	Is he still able to manage himself? Could you tell me more about the difficulties that he has been having?	Does he need additional help with any of the following? – Dressing – Washing – Toileting – Ambulation	Does he need additional help with any of the following? – Finances – Shopping – Food preparation – Transportation
Risk assessment	Have there been any other concerns with regard to his behaviour of late?	Has he wandered out of the house previously? Has he ever got lost when he was out of the house?	Has he been aggressive verbally or physically at home? Has he accidentally hurt himself recently?

Common pitfalls:

a. Failure to empathize with the caregiver at the start of the interview. Rapport building is essential in this station.
b. Failure to ask about frontal lobe symptoms such as disinhibited behaviours, executive planning and organization, and mood changes.
c. Failure to ask about risky behaviours.

STATION 50
COGNITIVE
ASSESSMENT

Information to candidates:

Name of patient: Mr Burd

Mr Burd has been referred by his GP to the specialist memory clinic. His son, Joseph, reports that his father has been having difficulties with his memory for the past year.

Task: Please assess for specific lobar deficits and general cognitive functioning.

Outline of station:

You are Joseph, the son of Mr Burd. You noted that your father's memory has been declining over the past year. He is having problems with an immediate recall of information, and at times, he cannot recall his distant relatives. Whilst he can still care for himself, you noticed that he had some personality changes in the last six months. He could be disinhibited at times. He has a long-standing history of poorly controlled blood pressure and diabetes mellitus. Five years ago, he had a minor cerebrovascular event. He has been maintained on lifelong aspirin treatment since. You understand that the psychiatrist is going to perform a series of examinations to evaluate the functioning of the different parts of his brain.

CASC Construct Table:

The CASC Construct Table is formatted such that candidates would be able adequately to cover both the range and depth of the assessment required in this station.

Starting off: "Hello, I am Dr Melvyn, one of the psychiatrists from the mental health unit. I understand from your GP that you have been having some memory issues. I am going to ask you to perform some tasks to assess the different parts of your brain. Some of these tasks are easy, and some tasks are difficult. Please try your best to perform."			
General cognition	Before we begin, could I check whether you have any visual or hearing impairments? Can you see and hear clearly?	Do you know where we are now? What level are we on? Which part of the country is this? What is the greater country that we are in?	Do you know what time it is now? Do you know what year this is? Can you tell me what season, month, day, and date today?

DOI: 10.1201/9781003313113-50

Temporal lobe assessment	I will be asking you questions that test the functioning of the lower part of your brain. I would like you to remember three objects, which I will ask you to repeat immediately and five minutes later.	The three objects I'd like you to remember are "apple," "table," and "penny."	Can you repeat the three objects that I have told you? Who is the current Prime Minister in the UK? (Write "Close your eyes" on a piece of paper.) Could you please read this sentence and do what it says? (After five minutes) Could you tell me the three objects that I asked you to remember earlier?
Frontal lobe assessment	I be asking you questions that test the functioning of the front part of your brain. Could you tell me your understanding of this proverb, "A stitch in time saves nine?"	Can you tell me about the similarities between an apple and orange? (Alternatively, use a table and chair as an example.) Could you tell me what the average height of an Englishman is? Could you tell me the approximate distance between London and Manchester?	I would like you to say as many words as possible, starting with the letter F in one minute, without naming any names of people. Could we begin? Alternatively, I would like you to say as many animals as you can within one minute.
Parietal lobe assessment	I will be asking you questions that test the functioning of the upper part of your brain. I'd like you to tell me the answer when 7 is taken away from 100.	Please continue to take away seven from the answer obtained and continue doing this. (Correct answer: 93, 86, 79, 72, 65.)	Please show me your right index finger. Please use your left index finger to touch your nose. (Testing for finger agnosia.)
Concluding the assessment	Thank you for cooperating with me on these tasks. How do you think you have performed?	I would need some time to review your results, and we will inform you how you have done.	

Common pitfalls:

d. Failure to cover the range and depth of the station.

e. Failure to select appropriate tasks and adapt accordingly if this station is conducted virtually.

STATION 51
MILD COGNITIVE IMPAIRMENT (PATIENT MANAGEMENT)

Information to candidates:

Name of patient: Mr Hunter

Mr Hunter is a 75-year-old male who has been having increasing difficulties with his memory over the past six months. He has been misplacing things and sometimes gets confused and lost in a conversation. He decided to check in with his GP last week, who referred him to your specialized service for further assessment and management. You saw the patient, Mr Hunter, one week ago and assessed him to have mild cognitive impairment. His wife is here today and wishes to speak to you.

Task: Please speak to Mrs Hunter and explain the diagnosis. Please also discuss with her your treatment plans for Mr Hunter. It would be best if you also addressed all her concerns and expectations.

Outline of station:

You are the wife of Mr Hunter. You understand that the psychiatrist has seen him and diagnosed him accordingly. You wish to know more about the assessment and the clinical diagnosis. When you're being told that your husband has mild cognitive impairment, you need to ask the candidate whether this is like dementia. You are concerned about whether your husband can live independently now that he has been diagnosed with mild cognitive impairment. In addition, you want to know more about the course and the prognosis of having such a diagnosis. You wonder whether your husband would benefit from the usage of anti-dementia drugs. You also wish to know how else you could help him and fully support him now that he has mild cognitive impairment. You also want to know the relevant risk factors that might predispose someone to develop dementia.

CASC Construct Table:

The CASC Construct Table is formatted such that candidates would be able adequately to cover both the range and depth of the assessment required in this station.

DOI: 10.1201/9781003313113-51

Starting off: "Hello, I am Dr Melvyn, one of the psychiatrists from the mental health unit. I understand that you have some concerns about your husband, Mr Hunter. Could we have a chat about it?"			
Clarification of assessment and diagnosis	We spoke to your husband last week, and we understand that he has been having memory difficulties for quite a while. It must have been a difficult time for you.	We have performed some clinical assessment and memory testing. As part of the clinical assessment, we explored his orientation, checked for any language and communication difficulties and general functioning, and a risk assessment. We have also conducted a mini-mental state examination (MMSE). The scores showed that he is likely having mild cognitive impairment.	Have you heard about mild cognitive impairment before? Thanks for sharing with me your understanding of mild cognitive impairment.
Explanation of rationale for diagnosis of mild cognitive impairment	Mild cognitive impairment is different from that of dementia.	Individuals with mild cognitive impairments usually have mild cognitive deficits, short of that usually observed and described for dementia. They might have poor performance on memory testing.	However, very often, individuals with mild cognitive impairment are usually able to function independently at home and handle their everyday activities. Do you have any questions about his diagnosis?
Explain the course and prognosis	For individuals who age normally, around 15% of them might eventually get mild cognitive impairment.	The average conversion rate from mild cognitive impairment to dementia is around 5–10% per day.	
Explain pharmacological treatment	Based on the local guidelines, there is unfortunately no medication that has been recommended for the treatment of this disorder.	Suppose your husband has other underlying medical issues, such as hypertension. In that case, it might be ideal for him to be on medication to ensure that his underlying medical conditions are well controlled.	Control of his underlying medical conditions would be essential as they are risk factors that would increase his chances of developing dementia.

(Continued)

(Continued)

Explain non-pharmacological treatments	I'm sorry to inform you that there is currently no medication that is indicated for the treatment of this condition.	Besides medication, lifestyle modifications could help prevent your husband from developing dementia.	We recommend that he partakes in regular exercises and keeps himself physically and mentally active. It is also essential that he eat a healthy diet.
Address any other concerns	I know that I have shared quite a lot of information today. Can I offer you a leaflet from the Royal College about mild cognitive impairment for you to better understand his condition?	Do you have any other concerns now? Thanks for your question. There are many factors that might predispose one to develop dementia.	Common risk factors include that of age, having a lower education level, having a previous history of depression, and being female in gender.

Common pitfalls:

  a. Failure to address all the concerns of the relatives.
  b. Failure to establish rapport and gradually disseminate information/being too check-listed in information giving.

**If the station requires the candidate to take a history to come to a diagnosis of mild cognitive impairments, the following aspects ought to be covered:

  a. Exploration of memory difficulties
  b. Exploration of orientation and visuospatial dysfunction
  c. Exploration of language, communication, and recognition difficulties
  d. Exploration of functioning
  e. Risk assessment

Please remember to conduct an MMSE for an objective assessment of memory.

STATION 52
DELIRIUM (PATIENT MANAGEMENT)

Information to candidates:

Name of patient: Mr Tonelli

Mr Tonelli is a 75-year-old male who has been admitted to the medical ward for an altered mental state. According to the history given by the family, it was noted that he has been having a high fever for the past four days. He was noted to be confused as well. The medical team has done routine bloodwork as well as scans for him. The medical team has referred him to psychiatry as they are concerned that there might be a potential underlying psychiatric cause.

Task: Please speak to the team's consultant, sharing more about the likely diagnosis and the possible management options.

Outline of station:

You are Dr Ian Sturgess and you have heard from this newly admitted patient. You wish to find out from your trainee about the presenting complaints and his current working differential diagnosis. In addition, you hope the trainee could substantiate his claims for his proposed differential diagnosis. You will question the trainee about the necessary investigations that should be conducted. You wish to know more about the potential treatment for the patient as well. You expect the trainee to provide more information about how the patient could be managed in the current ward.

CASC Construct Table:

The CASC Construct Table is formatted so that candidates can adequately cover both the range and depth of the assessment required in this station.

Starting off: "Hello, I am Ian. Could I discuss the case I just saw with you and the team?"			
Formulation of case	Mr Tonelli is a 75-year-old gentleman who has been admitted to the inpatient unit and referred to psychiatry for acute changes in behaviour associated with a high temperature. I have spoken to him and his daughter.	He does not have any past psychiatric history or known family psychiatric history. In addition, he has no known past chronic medical illnesses. However, he has recently been seen by his GP.	He is staying with his wife and his daughter, his main caregivers.

(Continued)

DOI: 10.1201/9781003313113-52

(Continued)

Explain diagnosis and aetiology	Upon interviewing the patient, I note that he has features suggestive of a likely ongoing delirium episode. He was inattentive when I conversed with him. He was confused and not orientated to time, place, and person. He also reports visual hallucinations.	I have checked the nursing charts and noted that he has sleep-wake disturbances as well. The nurses also observed that his consciousness tends to fluctuate, with him being alert sometimes during the day. He has had more behavioural issues at night. The observations I have noted are consistent with the collaborative history that his daughter has provided me with.	My differential diagnosis is of delirium. However, I cannot exclude the possibility of an underlying dementing process. Concerning the potential causes of delirium, there are likely many causes to be considered. For example, it might be due to an underlying infection, constipation, dehydration, pain, or due to drugs.
Explain investigations	I like to contact the GP to get more information about his recent assessment. In addition, I would like to know the medication that the GP might have started him on as well.	I understand that the medical team have ordered some basic bloodwork. I like to check for any abnormalities in the blood obtained. If a urine analysis has not been ordered, I would like to request for it as well.	Ideally, I would like to request some imaging studies if they have not been done as well.
Explain management plans—pharmacological	With regards to management, I would like to suggest that the patient would be best sited in a medical ward.	If the diagnosis is indeed delirium, medication could be started to treat the underlying cause (such as infection).	If he does have disturbing behaviours, I would not recommend that the team commence him immediately on psychotropic medication. Instead, non-pharmacological measures should be tried first.
Explain management plans—non-pharmacological	It is essential to optimize the environment and nursing care for the patient. It would be advisable for the patient to have a consistent nurse caring for his needs.	The nurse could help to provide regular re-orientation to the environment, which would be helpful for the patient.	Only in circumstances where non-pharmacological measures, such as reassurance, fails should psychotropic medication be considered. Usually, antipsychotics like haloperidol and quetiapine could be considered.

Explain prognosis	With regards to the prognosis of the condition, it is very much dependent on the underlying aetiological causes of the delirium process.	Usually, with adequate treatment, the delirium will clear up in around two to three weeks.	Do you have other questions for me?

Common pitfalls:

a. Failure to cover the range and depth of information required for the station.

b. Failure to determine whether there are any underlying cognitive issues.

In the event this station requires the candidate to elicit a history from the caregiver prior to the discussion of the case with the consultant psychiatrist, the following questions could be asked to elicit the core symptoms of delirium:

1. Are there times in the day in which you noticed that he is less confused?
2. Is he aware of his surroundings? Can he still recognize his caregivers? Does he know roughly what time of the day it is when you ask him?
3. Apart from the confusion you have mentioned, does he seem to be more sensitive to environmental changes? Or is he more inattentive and quieter than usual?

Information to candidates:

Name of patient: Mr Brush

Mr Brush is a 65-year-old male brought into the emergency services today by his son. Over the past two weeks, his son has noted that his father has had increasingly strange behaviours. He has been more irritable in his mood and has not been sleeping well. Despite the lack of sleep, he is still capable of helping with the family business. Over the last three days, his son has found out from his mother that his father has withdrawn £60,000 from his account to invest in a new property. His son is very concerned about this sudden change in behaviour. Your colleague in the emergency services has done some basic blood tests for him, which were all normal. An imaging study has been done, and it has been normal as well.

Task: Please speak to Mr Brush and take a history to come to a diagnosis. Please also perform a mental state examination.

Outline of station:

You are Mr Brush, and you are unsure why you have been brought to the emergency services. You feel perfectly well, and you have already refused to see the medical doctor previously. You turn irritable when being told that you need to see a psychiatrist. You will tell the psychiatrist that there is absolutely nothing wrong with you. You insist that the psychiatrist completes his evaluation fast as you have a lot of plans. You withdrew £60,000 from your bank account three days ago. You invested in a new property, and you have plans to distribute the rest of the money to the local charity service. You have not been sleeping well, but it does not concern you as your energy levels are superb. You shared that you have been granted special rights by the royal family and cannot be involuntarily admitted. You hear the Royal Family speaking to you at times. You do not have any thoughts of harming yourself or others.

CASC Construct Table:

The CASC Construct Table is formatted such that candidates would be able adequately to cover both the range and depth of the assessment required in this station.

DOI: 10.1201/9781003313113-53

Starting off: "Hello, I am Dr Melvyn, one of the psychiatrists from the mental health unit. I understand that your son brought you in today. Could we have a chat?"				
Eliciting core manic symptoms	How have you been feeling in your mood? If I were to ask you to rate your mood on a scale from 1 to 10, what score would you give your mood now? Have others commented that you have been more irritable recently?	How has your energy level been? How has your sleep been? Are you still as energetic as ever despite the decreased amount of sleep? How has your appetite been?	Are you able to think clearly? Do you feel that there are many thoughts racing through your mind at any moment?	How long have you been feeling this way for?
Eliciting grandiose delusional beliefs and challenging beliefs	It seems to me that you feel that you are specially chosen. Could you tell me more?	Are there any special powers or abilities that you have that others do not have? Could you tell me more about it?	Could there be other explanations for why you have all these symptoms/ special abilities? Could it be because you have been unwell?	Do you feel increasingly more confident about yourself recently?
Eliciting hallucinations in all other modalities, eliciting thought disorders, eliciting passivity experiences	**Auditory hallucinations** Do you hear sounds or voices that others do not hear? How many voices could you hear? Are they as clear as our current conversation? What do they say?	**Second-person auditory hallucinations** Do they speak directly to you? Can you give me some examples of what they have been saying to you?	**Third-person auditory hallucinations** Do they refer to you as "he" or "she," much like a third person? Do they comment on your actions? Do they give you orders or commands as to what to do?	How do you feel when you hear them? Could there be any alternative explanation for these experiences that you have been having? Do you feel that your thoughts are being interfered with by an external force? Do you feel in control of your own actions and emotions?

(Continued)

(Continued)

Risk assessment—risk of excessive spending, intimacy, self-harm, violence	Have you engaged in any activities recently that might be dangerous? By that, I mean, have you been involved with the police recently?	Have you been spending more money than usual?	Have you been recently involved in: – Any intimate relationships with others? – Any protected sexual activity?	Have you been so troubled by all these that you have entertained thoughts of ending your life? Have you got into trouble with others around you?
Impact and coping mechanisms	How have you been coping with all these?	Have you made use of any substances, such as alcohol, to help you cope?	What about street drugs?	

Common pitfalls:

  a. Failure to elicit core manic symptoms from patient/failure to cover the range and depth of the station.

  b. Failure to perform a complete risk assessment.

STATION 54 ELDERLY MANIA (PATIENT MANAGEMENT)

Information to candidates:

Name of patient: Mr Brush

Mr Brush is a 65-year-old male brought into the emergency services today by his son. Over the past two weeks, his son has noted that his father has had increasingly strange behaviours. He has been more irritable in his mood and has not been sleeping well. Despite the lack of sleep, he is still capable of helping with the family business. Over the last three days, his son has found out from his mother that his father has withdrawn £60,000 from his account to invest in a new property. His son is very concerned about this sudden change in behaviour. Your colleague in the emergency services has done some basic blood tests for him, which were all normal. An imaging study has been done, and it has been normal as well. You have seen Mr Brush in the previous station. His wife is here and wishes to know more about what has been wrong with him.

Task: Please speak to Mrs Brush and discuss the most probable diagnosis for her husband. Please also discuss your management plan with her and address all her concerns and expectations.

Outline of station:

You are Mr Brush's wife, Lydia, and you are very concerned about what has been wrong with your husband. You want to know his diagnosis after the psychiatrist has seen him. If the psychiatrist tells you that he has mania, you appear surprised and want to know why this diagnosis has been given. Given the acute changes in behaviour, you want to know whether this could be an acute confusion state. You want to know what the psychiatrist would recommend in terms of further management—should he be hospitalized? You appeared very concerned about hospitalization, as your husband will not be amenable to staying in the hospital. If the psychiatrist mentioned more about using the Mental Health Act to detain your husband, you appeared very concerned. You wish to know whether you could give consent on his behalf. You hope that the psychiatrist will keep you updated throughout the entire hospitalization.

CASC Construct Table:

The CASC Construct Table is formatted such that candidates would be able to cover adequately both the range and depth of the assessment required in this station.

DOI: 10.1201/9781003313113-54

Starting off: "Hello, I am Dr Melvyn, one of the psychiatrists from the mental health unit. Thanks for coming today. I have assessed your husband, and I hope we can have a chat to address all the concerns you have."			
Explanation of Diagnosis	I have spoken to your husband to understand more about the circumstances leading to the current admission. I have also performed a mental state examination.	I understand it has been difficult for you over the past week. It seemed to me that your husband most likely has mania with psychotic symptoms. Have you heard of mania or bipolar disorder before?	Other possibilities could include an acute confusion state or a drug-induced manic episode. However, these seemed to be less likely given that his routine blood screens and drug screen seemed to be normal. In addition, the imaging study conducted has been normal.
Clarification of diagnosis	It is quite likely that your husband has a manic episode. This is because he has some symptoms consistent with a manic episode, such as having flights of ideas, being more circumstantial in speech and having more paranoid ideations. Sometimes, when patients are in a manic state, they tend to be more irritable as well.	Can I check with you whether your husband has a previous psychiatric history? Does he have any other chronic medical conditions we need to know? (Or) If he has a chronic medical condition, has he been on consistent follow-ups with any specific doctors?	Would you mind if we obtain further information from the regular doctor that he has been following up with?
Management	I understand that your family has been having difficulties managing your husband's behaviour over the past week. We would like to recommend a short period of inpatient observation and management.	The aim of an inpatient admission is largely for us to continue observation of his mental state and to commence treatment. We hope the inpatient observation will help minimize the associated risks. Likely, your husband will also benefit from the input of our multidisciplinary team.	We could try pharmacological treatment using medication like lithium and/or antipsychotics (like olanzapine) to help stabilize his mood. Unfortunately, if he is not responsive to or even intolerant to this combination, electroconvulsive therapy might be indicated.

Other concerns and expectations	Do you have any other concerns about how we are going to manage your husband? I hear you are concerned about his not wanting to be admitted.	Given the acute change in mental state and the risk involved, we could detain him involuntarily under the Mental Health Act. I'm sorry we have to resort to doing this. Unfortunately, if he is detained under the Mental Health Act, it is not possible for relatives to give proxy consent.	I hear that you are very concerned about your husband's concern. Please rest assured that my team and I will keep you updated about his clinical progression during his inpatient stay. Please feel free to contact us and make an appointment to meet us should you have further queries.

Common pitfalls:

a. Failure to consider alternative differential diagnosis and explain alternatives conceptualized.
b. Failure to explain why it is most likely mania given the history obtained and the mental state examination was done previously.
c. Failure to address concerns adequately.
d. Failure to explain in detail management plans for elderly mania.

TOPIC III
CHILD PSYCHIATRY

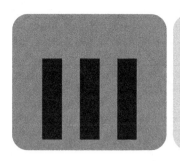

STATION 55
ADHD HISTORY TAKING

Information to candidates:

Name of patient: David Flowers

The local GP has referred David, a 5-year-old boy, to your service for further assessment. He is here today together with his mother, Mrs Flowers. It was noted in the referring memo that David has been having a lot of difficulties both at home and in school, and his mother is very concerned.

Task: Please speak to Mrs Flowers, David's mother, to elicit more information about him, looking for features suggestive of a childhood disorder. Please also consider other associated comorbidities and rule them out in your history taking.

Outline of station:

You are Mrs Flowers, the mother of your son, David. He is 5 years old this year and has been having problematic behaviours both in school and at home. Both you and his teacher have noted that he is hyperactive and cannot sit still. He is inattentive most of the time. In addition, you are especially concerned about his impulsive actions. There was an occasion when he was almost involved in an accident as he dashed across the traffic junction. There are no other abnormal behaviours that you have noted. He has not got himself into any major conduct problems, and he can still handle the work expected of his academic level. His speech is normal. There is no family history of any psychiatric disorders.

CASC Construct Table:

The CASC Construct Table is formatted such that candidates would be able adequately to cover both the range and depth of the assessment required in this station.

DOI: 10.1201/9781003313113-55

Starting off: "Hello, I am Dr Melvyn, one of the psychiatrists from the mental health unit. I understand that you came to see us today as you have some concerns about your son, David. Would you mind telling me more?"			
Background information	I understand from your GP that you have been having some difficulties with managing David. Could you tell me when this first started?	Would you mind sharing with me the difficulties you have been facing? I'm sorry to be hearing all this. Are these behaviours only limited to school? Are there other occasions to which you have noticed such behaviours as well?	In what way do you think David is different from a child typical of his age? Thanks for sharing your concerns with me. I hope to be of help. Could we spend the next few minutes understanding more about the difficulties?
Eliciting hyperactivity symptoms (mnemonic to remember: WORST) —Waiting in queue is difficult —Outburst —Restless —Squirms when seating —Talks excessively	You mentioned that David is always on the go? Could you give me some examples?	Is he able to remain in his seat when he is at school? Does he tend to squirm when sitting? What happens if you are out with David for a family meal?	Are there times at which he climbs on furniture? Is he able to wait in turn in a queue? Does he tend to talk excessively when others are talking?
Eliciting inattention symptoms (mnemonic to remember: SOLID) —Start tasks but do not finish —Organization impairment —Lose things easily —Inattentive —Distractable	I understand that one of your other concerns is that he seemed to be inattentive. What has his teacher reported when he is in school?	Have you noticed similar problems when he is at home? Can he concentrate on tasks that you have asked him to do? Do you find that he is easily distracted?	Are there times when he noticed that he seemed quite forgetful and kept misplacing things? Is he able to organize things at home or in school?

Eliciting Impulsiveness symptoms (mnemonic to remember: FAIL) —Fidget —Answer before the teacher finishes questions —Impulsive —Loud	I am very concerned to hear about what he has done previously (dashing out onto the roads). Is that an isolated incident?	Have there been other similar episodes in which you are concerned about his safety?	Did his teacher report similar incidents in school? Has his teacher reported that he tends to answer before the teacher finishes questioning? Did his teacher ever mention that he always has problems waiting for his turn?
Consideration of other comorbidities	I'm sorry to know how tough things have been for you concerning managing his difficult behaviours. Does anyone in the family have any previous psychiatric history?	Besides the symptoms you have reported, have you noticed any unusual movements that David has? Does he happen to have any language problems? Is he able to play with the other children? Is he able to reciprocate when you show your affection towards him?	Could you tell me more about his school performance? Has he got into any conduct problems in school or with the police? How has his mood been? Is he still able to enjoy doing the things he used to enjoy doing? Thanks for sharing with me. I am hopeful our team could help your son, David, with his condition.

Common pitfalls:

a. Failure to ask sufficient questions to cover the range and depth of the information required to make a diagnosis of ADHD or hyperkinetic disorder.

b. Failure to ask questions about and exclude other possible comorbid conditions.

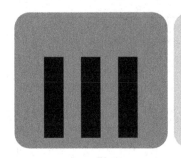

STATION 56
ADHD (PATIENT MANAGEMENT)

Information to candidates:

Name of patient: David Flowers

The local GP has referred David, a 5-year-old boy, to your service for further assessment. He is here today together with his mother, Mrs Flowers. It was noted in the referring memo that David has been having a lot of difficulties both at home and in school, and his mother is very concerned. You have spoken to the mother, obtained a school report, and done some psychometric testing for David. It has been established that David has a diagnosis of ADHD. His mother has booked another appointment today as she has some concerns about the diagnosis. She wants to have more information about the medication that might be started. As David is her oldest child, she is very concerned that the rest of her children will get ADHD as well.

Task: Please speak to Mrs Flowers, David's mother, explain the diagnosis, and address all her concerns and expectations.

Outline of station:

You are Mrs Flowers, the mother of David. You heard that the team had diagnosed David with ADHD. You have only heard about ADHD from the media. You want the doctor to explain to you in a simple manner what ADHD really is. You are curious about the condition and wish to know more. You wonder whether you are responsible for David having ADHD. You like to know what the other causes of ADHD are. You understand that treatment is available. If the doctor proposes some medication, you appear to be very concerned and want to know the exact side effects. You have concerns about the major side effects of growth suppression. As you have other children, you wonder at the likelihood of them having ADHD. You also wonder whether there are blood tests that could confirm the diagnosis. You have heard in the news that a special diet might be helpful. You are curious as to whether you could try some sort of special diet as well for David.

CASC Construct Table:

The CASC Construct Table is formatted so that candidates can adequately cover both the range and depth of the assessment required in this station.

DOI: 10.1201/9781003313113-56

Starting off: "Hello, I am Dr Melvyn, one of the psychiatrists from the mental health unit. I understand that you came to see us today as you have some concerns about your son, David. Would you mind telling me more?"			
Explanation of diagnosis	Thanks for coming today. I understand that you are concerned about our diagnosis for David.	Yes, you're right that the team diagnosed him with ADHD. Have you heard about ADHD before? What is your understanding of ADHD?	ADHD is a terminology commonly used in the US. In the UK, the disorder is termed hyperkinetic disorder.
Clarification of symptoms and underlying aetiology	Children diagnosed with this condition tend to have three symptoms: hyperactivity, inattention, and impulsiveness. Hyperkinetic disorder is common in the UK, affecting 1.7% of all school-going children. It tends to be more common in males as compared to females. While I understand your concerns about the diagnosis, there are effective treatments for this condition. As we will share later, medication can help with the core symptoms.	Unfortunately, no specific blood test or brain imaging would guide us towards the diagnosis. We have diagnosed David with ADHD based on the history you have provided us with and the collaborative history we have obtained from the school. In addition, we administered the Corner scale for David, and he was in the abnormal range on the scale.	With regard to your concerns about the causation of the disorder, multiple factors may be responsible. If there is a family history of the disorder, there is a two-fold increment in the risk of the child having the disorder. Disturbances in the normal brain chemicals, as well as infections or problems during pregnancy, might predispose individuals towards ADHD as well.
Explain management (pharmacological)	I'm sorry to inform you that David has ADHD. I am hopeful that our team can help him with his condition. Some medications are available to help him. The most used medication is methylphenidate, a stimulant. Have you heard about it before?	Like all medications, methylphenidate does have its side effects. Before we start any medication, we need to perform a full physical examination, measure his blood pressure, and do a heart tracing. We will also measure his baseline height and weight. We will commence the lowest dose and adjust the medication in accordance with his response to the medication.	Methylphenidate works by normalizing the amounts of certain chemicals in the brain. It helps to make the child calmer and more focused with increased attention. The most common side effects are a reduction in appetite, weight loss, headaches, difficulties with sleep, and irritable mood. If he experiences any rare side effects, such as shortness of breath, allergic reactions, or heart problems, please bring him back for an urgent review.

(Continued)

(Continued)

			The most common long-term side effect is growth suppression; hence, we make it a point to measure his height and weight during each clinic review. Some individuals might present with tics or have abnormal facial movements following the use of methylphenidate—if this is the case, we will consider other medication (non-stimulants).
Explain management (non-pharmacological)	Apart from medication, there are also other non-pharmacological methods that we could use to help David.	It is essential that you are referred to educational programmes to learn more about ADHD, its management, and coping strategies.	We could also refer David to see a psychologist to be engaged in behaviour therapy. Environmental modifications, such as placing the child in the front row of the class, may help to reduce distractions.
Address concerns	I know that we have discussed quite a lot today. Do you have any questions for me?	Existing research has not proven that a special diet will be helpful for children.	As the hyperkinetic disorder is a heritable condition, there is an increased chance that your other children might develop the disorder.

Common pitfalls:

a. Failure to explain ADHD concisely.
b. Failure to address the mother's concerns about stimulants and explain the most common side effects. It is important to highlight some of the rare side effects and mention the consideration of non-stimulants if the child presents with tics.
c. Failure to address its effects on other children.

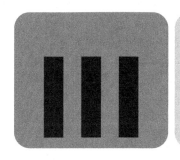

STATION 57
CONDUCT DISORDER
(HISTORY TAKING)

Information to candidates:

Name of patient: Samson Hellers

The school counsellor has requested an early appointment with the child psychiatrist for Samson Hellers, a 14-year-old male. He has been physically threatening his school peers and recently involved in a theft. The school feels that he would benefit from further assessment and management. His mother, Mrs Hellers, has been informed of the referral and is with her son today.

Task: Please speak to Mrs Hellers, Samson's mother, and take a history to arrive at an appropriate diagnosis. Please obtain other relevant personal histories from his mother as well.

Outline of station:

You are Mrs Hellers, Samson's mother, and you have heard about his increasingly difficult behaviour in school. You're very concerned to learn that your son has been involved in a recent theft case in school. You hope this is not because he is mixing with bad company. You have noted that since he was young, he has been cruel towards animals. When he was in junior school, you received feedback from his teachers, who said that he is physically aggressive and has been threatening to harm his peers. Now that he is in high school, you understand that he has also frequently missed school. You hope that this is not because you are struggling to make ends meet and cannot provide your son with quality time and care, given that you need to work long hours. Your husband is currently in prison following a grievous crime that he committed three years ago. You hope that the psychiatrist can help your son with regard to his behaviour issues as you hope that he will not end up in a similar state to your husband.

CASC Construct Table:

The CASC Construct Table is formatted so that candidates can adequately cover both the range and depth of the assessment required in this station.

DOI: 10.1201/9781003313113-57

Starting off: "Hello, I am Dr Melvyn, one of the psychiatrists from the mental health unit. I understand that the school counsellor has some concerns for your son, Samson, and hence has arranged this appointment. Could we have a chat about your concerns?"		
Clarification of history	Thank you for being here today. I understand that it must have been a difficult time for you. Could you share with me more about your concerns pertaining to Samson?	How long have you noted Samson to be having these difficult behaviours? (Or) Do you remember when all these difficult behaviours first started?	Would you say that Samson has violated rules in the past 12 months and been aggressive, destructive, and deceitful? Or in the past six months, has he violated any rules, been aggressive, been destructive or been deceitful?
Specific symptoms (towards adults)	Has he had frequent arguments with adults/ yourself? Does he defy set rules or any other specific requests set by adults/yourself?	Has he stayed out late at night without your permission?	
Specific symptoms (towards other people)	How has he been around other people? Have you noticed that he has been annoying them intentionally? Does he tend to blame others for his own mistakes?	Has he gotten into any fights with others? If he has, has he used any weapons to harm others? Has he exhibited any cruelty towards others or even to animals?	Do you know if he has forced others into sexual activities?
Specific symptoms (towards objects or properties)	Has there been any occasion on which he has deliberately destroyed properties?	My understanding is that he has been recently involved in a theft. Could you tell me more about it? Has he been involved in any other crimes previously?	Has there been any time when he has run away from home?
Eliciting predisposing risk factors	Could I check whether there is a family history of any psychiatric-related disorder? Could you tell me more about your husband? Do you know if he has had conduct problems previously whilst he was in school? Has he been involved in any other crimes?	Is there a history of substance usage in the family (such as alcohol)? How are the finances in the family?	Were there any problems with Samson when he was growing up? Was there anyone who was harsh to him or had to resort to severe physical and verbal punishment to deal with his difficult behaviours?

Ruling out comorbidity	How has Samson's mood been in the past month or so? Have you realized that he is losing interest in things he used to enjoy? Would you say that Samson has been more anxious lately?	Can Samson focus on tasks that you assign him to do? Is he always on the go (hyperactive)? Does he have any learning difficulties? How is his current academic performance?	Are you aware whether Samson is using any alcohol or street drugs now?

Common pitfalls:

a. Failure to cover the range and depth required for the station.
b. Failure to elicit predisposing risk factors that would contribute towards the child developing conduct disorder.
c. Failure to rule out comorbidities.

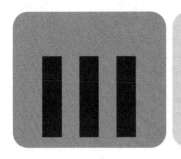

Information to candidates:

Name of patient: Mrs Young

Mrs Young has been having some concerns about her 4-year-old son, Jonathan. She feels that his language abilities are limited and not on par with the rest of the normal children of his age. In addition, she noticed that her child cannot reciprocate her affection at times and has very minimal eye contact, even towards the rest of the family members. Her local GP has recommended that she seek help from a child psychiatrist for Jonathan, and she is here today to share her concerns.

Task: Please speak to Mrs Young and elicit more history to come to a possible diagnosis. Please also take other necessary personal and developmental histories pertinent to the formulation of the eventual diagnosis.

Outline of station:

You are Mrs Young, and Jonathan is your only child. Before he was 3 years old, you had already noted that he had delayed language abilities. You also noticed that Jonathan has abnormal reciprocal social interaction. He has poor eye contact and cannot play with the other children at the playgroup. He is not able to show his affection towards you. He does not usually play with his toys in the usual way, like how the other children would play. He tends to be preoccupied with parts of the toys instead. Thus far, you have not noticed any other additional problems, such as sleeping or eating disturbances, aggression, or self-injury behaviour.

CASC Construct Table:

The CASC Construct Table is formatted so that candidates can adequately cover both the range and depth of the assessment required in this station.

DOI: 10.1201/9781003313113-58

Starting off: "Hello, I am Dr Melvyn, one of the psychiatrists from the mental health unit. I understand that your local GP has arranged for you to see us as you have some concerns about your child, Jonathan. Could we have a chat about this?"		
Clarification of the history and onset of symptoms	I'm sorry to hear about the difficulties that you have been facing with Jonathan. I hope to understand the situation better so we can help your child.	Could you tell me approximately at what age you first noticed these behavioural changes? (Or) Did you first notice these behavioural difficulties when Jonathan was younger than 3 years old?	Since then, how have things progressed?
Presence of abnormal reciprocal social interactions	Is Jonathan able to make eye contact with you or your family members when you speak to him?	Is he able to reciprocate your affection when you hug him?	Is he able to make friends with other children? Is he able to share toys and play together with other children?
Presence of abnormal communication	Could you tell me more about his language abilities? Do you know what his language difficulties are?	Is he even able to initiate and sustain a normal conversation with you? Does he tend to make use of or say the same phrase repetitively?	Have you noticed whether he tends to repeat spoken words others have said? Does he keep repeating what he has just said?
Presence of restricted, stereotyped, and repetitive behaviour	Have you noticed anything odd when Jonathan is allowed to play by himself? Does he seem to be preoccupied with parts of certain toys?	Does he play with his toys in the same way that other children play? Could you tell me more about his interests? Does he tend to do anything repeatedly/follow rituals?	Do you think he is able to adapt to changes in the environment? Have you noticed whether Jonathan has any other characteristic body movements (such as hand flapping and body rocking)? Is he sensitive to touch?
Other psychiatric comorbidities	How has his mood been? Is he still able to keep up with his interests? How have his sleep and appetite been?	Are there any specific things that Jonathan is afraid of?	Has there been any aggressive behaviour? Has there been any self-injurious behaviour?
Developmental history	Could you tell me more about your pregnancy? Were there any complications prior to, during, or after the pregnancy and delivery?	I like to enquire more about his developmental milestones. For example, do you remember when he first started to smile, turn over, crawl, sit, and walk?	Are there any other developmental issues I need to know of? Does he have any hearing impairment? Does he have a previous history of epilepsy? Has he been diagnosed with any genetic condition, such as fragile X syndrome?

Common pitfalls:

   a. Failure to cover the range and depth of the information required to confirm the diagnosis of autistic disorder.

   b. Failure to elicit information about developmental history.

**Although this is a history taking station, it is important to demonstrate empathy towards the parent, who may be distressed, worried, and anxious.

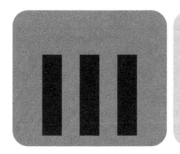

STATION 59
EARLY-ONSET
PSYCHOSIS (HISTORY
TAKING)

Information to candidates:

Name of patient: Paula Makeson

The local GP has referred Paula Makeson, as her parents feel that she has not been her usual self. They are apprehensive that there might be something wrong with her mental health as her grades have been declining, and she is also reluctant to go to school.

Task: Please speak to Paula Makeson in this station and elicit a history to come to a possible diagnosis. Please perform a relevant mental state examination.

Outline of station:

You are Paula Makeson, and you have been to the GP with your parents last week. You've been told that you needed to see a child psychiatrist. For the past two months, you have not been going to school as you feel that your friends are all talking about you behind your back. Despite you feeling this way, you have not confronted them about this matter. Your grades have declined as well. You do not hear voices and do not have any other strange experiences. You have tried cannabis once (which your parents are not aware of) when your close friends ask you to try. You have no thoughts of self-harm or suicide.

CASC Construct Table:

The CASC Construct Table is formatted so that candidates can adequately cover both the range and depth of the assessment required in this station.

Starting off: "Hello, I am Dr Melvyn, one of the psychiatrists from the mental health unit. I understand that your local GP has arranged for you to see me. Could we have a chat?"			
Eliciting core delusion and other delusional beliefs	I understand that there have been some difficulties at school. Could you tell me more? I'm sorry to hear that you have been feeling this way. It must have been a very difficult time for you.	How do you know that your friends are talking about you? Could there be any other alternative explanations for the way they behave?	Do you feel that other people out there are trying to harm you in any other way? Do you feel that you have some special powers or abilities? Do you feel that certain things have a special meaning for you?

(Continued)

DOI: 10.1201/9781003313113-59

(Continued)

Hallucinations	Auditory hallucinations Do you hear sounds or voices that others do not hear? How many voices could you hear? Are they as clear as our current conversation? What do they say?	Second-person auditory hallucinations Do they speak directly to you? Can you give me some examples of what they have been saying to you? **Third-person auditory hallucinations** Do they refer to you as "he" or "she," much like a third person? Do they comment on your actions? Do they give you orders or commands as to what to do? How do you feel when you hear them?	Visual hallucinations Do you see things which other people do not see? Could there be any alternative explanation for these experiences that you have been having?
Thought disorders	**Thought interference** Do you feel that your thoughts are being interfered with? Who do you think is doing this? **Thought insertion** Do you have thoughts in your head that you feel are not your own? Where do you think these thoughts come from?	**Thought broadcasting** Do you feel that your thoughts are being broadcasted such that others would know what you are thinking?	**Thought withdrawal** Do you feel that your thoughts are being taken away from your head by some external force?
Passivity experiences	Do you feel in control of your own actions and emotions?	Do you feel that someone or something is trying to control you? Who or what do you think this would be?	Other related symptoms: Do you find it tough to be motivated in things which you do? Have there been any changes in your self-care? (Screen for the presence of negative symptoms.)
Impact on mood and coping	Has this affected your mood in any way? Are you still interested in things you used to enjoy?	I understand that this must be a difficult time for you. How have you been coping?	Have you made use of any substances, such as alcohol, to help you cope? What about street drugs?
Risk assessment	Are you so troubled that you have entertained thoughts of ending your life?	What plans have you made?	Have you made any plans to approach those speaking about you?

Common pitfalls:

a. Failure to explore other delusional beliefs.
b. Failure to cover the range and the depth of the task required for the station.
c. Failure to screen for negative symptoms—such as the lack of motivation, self-care, poor attention, and lack of interest.
d. Failure to perform a comprehensive risk assessment (risk assessment needs to consider risk towards oneself as well as a risk towards others).

**Studies have shown that adolescents with early-onset psychosis tend to have worse premorbid functioning during late adolescence and are more likely to present with bizarre behaviour and primary negative symptoms. (Ballageer T, Malla A, Manchanda R, Takhar J, Haricharan R. Is adolescent-onset first-episode psychosis different from adult onset? *J Am Acad Child Adolesc Psychiatry.* 2005 Aug;44(8):782–9. doi: 10.1097/01.chi.0000164591.55942.ea. PMID: 16034280.)

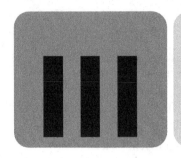

Information to candidates:

Name of patient: Paula Makeson

Paula Makeson has been referred by the local GP in view that she has not been her usual self. You have seen her, taken a history, and performed a mental state examination. During the clinical interview and mental state examination, you have elicited some positive symptoms, namely, that of visual and auditory hallucinations and paranoid ideations towards her classmates. In addition, she has had difficulties with her academic studies and has been neglecting self-care. You have a working diagnosis of what she has and have some interim management plans for her.

Task: Please speak to Dr Jan Cullen, the child psychiatrist on call, and discuss the differential diagnosis and your management plans for the patient.

Outline of station:

You are Dr Jan Cullen, the child psychiatrist on call. You understand that your core trainee has just seen Paula Makeson. You need to know more about the case and are keen to hear from the core trainee their formulation of the case. You need the trainee to tell you what possible differentials they are considering and their management plans in accordance with the differentials that they have suggested. You need the trainee to tell you specifically how they would manage the patient in the acute and long-term settings.

CASC Construct Table:

The CASC Construct Table is formatted so that candidates can adequately cover the range and depth of the assessment required in this station.

DOI: 10.1201/9781003313113-60

Starting off: "Hello, I am Melvyn, the on-call trainee. I have seen Paula Makeson and have performed a mental state examination of the patient. Could I present my assessment and my management plans to you?"			
Summary of psychiatric formulation	I have spoken to Paula Makeson, a 17-year-old student. She has been isolating herself from school for the past 2 months as she has paranoid ideations towards her classmates. These ideations are of delusional intensity. In addition, she did report that she was experiencing both auditory and visual hallucinations. She reported that she has had difficulties with her academic work and have at times neglected her self-care.	She does not have any significant medical or past psychiatric history that I have taken note of. She does not have any family history of any psychiatric disorders.	With regards to her mental state, she appears neat and groomed. She maintains some eye contact during the interview. Her mood is not overtly low, and her affect is appropriate. She is relevant throughout the interview. She reports that she is troubled by visual hallucinations and second-person auditory hallucinations. She denies harbouring any suicidal or homicidal ideations.
Explain differential diagnosis	Could I go on to discuss the possible differential diagnosis that I have considered?	I'd like to consider the possibility of her having first-episode psychosis. This is because she has both positive and negative symptoms.	The other differentials that I like to consider and exclude are depression with psychotic symptoms and substance-induced psychosis. The differential of depression with psychotic symptoms is less likely as she does not have mood-congruent hallucinations. With regards to substance-induced psychosis, she denies any substance use, but we need to perform further investigations to exclude this.

(Continued)

(Continued)

Explain general management (pharmacological)	Regarding management, I suggest that we do the necessary bloodwork to exclude an underlying organic aetiology. In addition, a toxicology screen would be essential to exclude the possibility of this being drug-induced psychosis.	Once we have ascertained that this is indeed first-episode psychosis, based on the NICE guidelines, we could commence her on a low dose of antipsychotics. My preference would be to commence her on an atypical antipsychotic as it is associated with lesser side effects.	An example of an antipsychotic that I would consider will be that of Risperidone. I will psycho-educate her about the medication and explain all the side effects. I will adjust the medication dosage in accordance with how she responds to the initiation of the medication.
Explain management (non-pharmacological)	Apart from medication, I'd like to suggest other alternatives to help Paula and her family. Providing education to Paula and her family about her condition and reinforcing compliance to medication will be essential.	In addition, the family needs to be educated about the relapse indicators so they could bring her back for an admission if needed. At times, psychological therapy such as cognitive behavioural therapy might be beneficial. I will closely monitor Paula's condition and will refer her to a psychologist when she is more settled in her mental state.	If there are highly expressed emotions within the family, I would like to recommend family therapy for the family as well.
Address consultant's concerns	I hope that I have adequately discussed how best we could help Paula. Are there any questions you have for me? I would like to manage Paula as an outpatient for now as there are no risk factors that I managed to elicit. However, she would benefit from engagement with the early psychosis intervention team. In the event that she presents with any risk (for example, risk of harm to herself or others), I will consider inpatient admission for her.	If she is not compliant with her medication, I would like to consider getting her more support in the community. This might involve having a community nurse doing home visitation. If she is still not compliant, I might consider speaking to the patient and the family about the commencement of a depot medication.	I am hoping she will respond to the antipsychotic we intend to start. Should she not respond to adequate trials of both typical and atypical antipsychotics, clozapine might be an option.

Common pitfalls:

a. Failure to cover the range and depth needed for the station (explain both pharmacological and non-pharmacological treatment needed).
b. Failure to discuss more getting the first-episode psychosis team involved.
c. Failure to address adequately the concerns raised by the consultant about outpatient monitoring, administration of a depot, and commencement of clozapine. It is essential to know the NICE guidelines about schizophrenia treatment to explain treatment options in this station.

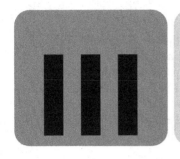

Information to candidates:

Name of patient: Annie Lloyd

You are the on-call core trainee and have been called to see a 15-year-old girl in the accident and emergency department as she has overdosed on 50 tablets of paracetamol tablets. The medics have done basic bloodwork for her and started her on medical management for her overdose. During the psychiatric clinical interview, the girl, Annie Lloyd, showed you a paper with the word "rape" on it when you asked her what her stressor was recently. She also pointed out the man in the waiting area (whom you know was her stepfather) when you asked who was involved.

Task: Please discuss the information you have obtained with the consultant on call.

Please discuss with the consultant how you wish to manage this case.

Outline of station:

The questions asked in the CASC grid will cover the outline of this station.

CASC Construct Table:

The CASC Construct Table is formatted so that candidates can adequately cover the range and depth of the assessment required in this station.

Starting off: "Hello, I am Melvyn, the on-call trainee. I have a patient in the emergency room, and I'd like to discuss this case with you. Could I proceed on?"			
Summary of the case	I have spoken to Annie Lloyd, a 15-year-old girl who has been admitted to the emergency department following an overdose on 50 tablets of paracetamol.	During the clinical interview, she was not willing and forthcoming about the circumstances that led her to overdose. She eventually showed me a paper with the word "rape" on it and pointed to her stepfather in the waiting area when I asked who was involved.	In view of the seriousness of the allegations, I have had to terminate the interview at that point, to avoid contamination of the information obtained from the child. I have asked a nurse to be with her for now, whilst I discuss this case with you.

DOI: 10.1201/9781003313113-61

Explain limitations	I am not able to obtain more information about the allegation, in view of my concerns about the possible contamination of the evidence. However, I have obtained sufficient information to evaluate her current suicide risk.	In addition, in view of the seriousness of the allegations, I have informed Annie, the child involved, that there is a need for me to break the confidentiality of the information.	I have clearly explained to her that I needed to share this information with my colleagues to ascertain the nature of the facts involved.
Acute management	Annie would require continued medical management given that she has just overdosed on many pills. I would like to offer her admission to the inpatient child medical ward for further observation and monitoring.	It is clear to me that she is still distressed by the circumstances that she has been in. I will inform my nurses to place her on suicide caution and, ideally, also recommend one-to-one nursing for her. I like to make an urgent referral to the social worker. In addition, I like to inform the child protection officer from the relevant agencies and the police as well.	I would have to inform her mother as her mother has parental responsibility over Annie. I'd like to briefly explain to her the current situation and advise her that a period of inpatient observation is essential for us to find out more about the allegation. I need to inform her mother that we need to restrict her stepfather's access regarding visitation. Given the circumstances involved, I need to ascertain from the mother whether there are other vulnerable individuals currently at home and advise her accordingly.

(Continued)

(Continued)

Intermediate and long-term management	I hope that the on-call consultant could discuss with the lead consultant in-charge of child abuse cases and a formal interview be conducted with the child.	In the intermediate short-term, the social worker or the police could offer an emergency protection order or a police protection order to ensure that the child is placed in a place of safety. If the allegations are ascertained to be true subsequently, they could help with facilitating an alternative accommodation for the child. In the event that the parents do not agree, a care order could be issued.	I'd like to recommend that the child be engaged with a counsellor for counselling services to deal with the emotional issues that have arisen due to the abuse. Other modalities of psychological therapy might also be helpful for the child.

Common pitfalls:

a. Failure to explain why the interview needs to be stopped once information pertaining to the sexual abuse has been shared.

b. Failure to explain in depth the recommended acute, intermediate, and long-term management plans.

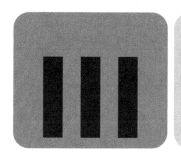

Information to candidates:

Name of patient: Amelia Smith

> You are the core trainee on call, and you have been asked to see Amelia Smith, a 15-year-old girl who has been brought into the accident and emergency department following a massive overdose of her mother's psychiatric medication. Her mother shared with the medical team that her daughter has been experiencing some difficulties at school. She is extremely distressed with her daughter's condition. The medical team has done the necessary blood works and have stabilized her condition. You have been asked to further evaluate Amelia Smith.

Task: Please speak to Amelia Smith to identify her reasons for her overdose and to perform an appropriate suicide risk assessment.

Outline of station:

> You are Amelia Smith, a 15-year-old girl who has just overdosed on all your mother's psychiatric medication. You come from a single-parent family, and your new school has been too much for you to handle. Because of your size, your peers in your new school have been calling you nasty names. There was an occasion on which they tried to lay hands on you after you argued with them. You have contemplated overdosing on medication for the past two weeks and have decided to go ahead today as you feel that life is no longer worth living, and you are too distressed by your experience in school. There is no one to whom you could share your problems, not even your mother, as she is busy working to make ends meet. You're willing to share the circumstances with the doctor, but you do not feel that sharing with the psychiatrist would help matters at school.

CASC Construct Table:

The CASC Construct Table is formatted so that candidates can adequately cover the range and depth of the assessment required in this station.

DOI: 10.1201/9781003313113-62

Starting off: "Hello, I am Dr Melvyn, one of the psychiatrists from the mental health unit. I have some information about why you have been admitted to the hospital. Could we have a chat about it?"		
Exploration of current attempts	I understand from the medical doctor that you have been admitted to the hospital following an overdose. I am sorry to hear that. It seems that things have been difficult for you. Could you take me through what has happened today? How long have you been thinking about overdosing? Where did you get those tablets? Did you write any last notes or letters to your loved ones prior to consuming all the tablets?	Could you tell me where you were when you took all those medicines? Was there anyone with you? (Or) If you were at home, did you take steps to ensure that no one would discover you? Did you take all the medicines at once? Did you take the medicines with any other substances? What was running through your mind when you took those tablets? Did you have thoughts of ending it all? How dangerous do you think taking that number of medicines would be? How did you feel after taking all the medicines? How were you discovered? Who brought you to the hospital?	Now that you are in hospital, do you regret that your overdose attempt was not successful? (Or) Are you remorseful about what you have done?
Exploration of underlying stressors	I understand that it has been a very difficult time for you. Could you share with me more about what has been bothering you?	(Or) Can you tell me what sort of things you have been bothered by? How have things been at home, in school or at work?	Do you have any relationship issues?
In-depth exploration of core stressors	I'm sorry to hear about the issue that has been troubling you. Could you tell me more about it? What have they done towards you? Have they called you names? Have they been physical against you? Have they done other things to cause you emotional hurt, such as spreading rumours about you?	How long has this been going on for you? How often does this happen in a week? Does this only happen in school? Do you have similar experiences out of school?	Did you manage to share with anyone more about this? How did your classmate respond when you told them about this? How did your teacher respond when you told her about this? Do you feel safe when you are in school/outside?

Other psychiatric comorbidities	Has this affected your mood in any way? Are you still interested in things you used to enjoy?	How have you been sleeping and eating?	Are you frequently bothered by flashbacks of the events that have happened? Are you bothered by nightmares in your sleep? Do you avoid school? Would you say that you have been feeling more on edge recently?
Risk assessment and coping mechanisms	Are you so troubled that you have entertained thoughts of ending your life? What plans have you made?	I understand that this must be a difficult time for you. How have you been coping?	Have you made use of any substances, such as alcohol, to help you cope? What about street drugs?

Common pitfalls:

a. Failure to perform a comprehensive suicide risk assessment.
b. Forgetting to ask about emotional bullying apart from verbal and physical bullying.
c. Detailed exploration of bullying (frequency and types of bullying, adult and peer response, locations, teacher perceptions and attitudes about bullying, aspects of the school or community that may support or help stop it, patient's perception of safety).

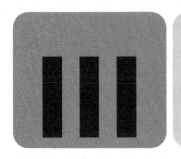

Information to candidates:

Name of patient: Joseph Bayers

Joseph Bayers is a 7-year-old male who has just started school. Sarah, Joseph's mother, has recently received feedback from his teachers that his academic performance in school is poor. Sarah has noted that over the past month, she has noted that there were many nights to which Joseph wets his bed. She is increasingly concerned about this. She has brought Joseph for an evaluation by the local GP, who has referred him to see you.

Task: Please speak to Sarah, Joseph's mother, and elicit more history about the current presenting problem, aiming to establish and arrive at a diagnosis.

Outline of station:

You are Sarah, Joseph's mother, and you are quite concerned about your son's condition. He has just recently started school, and you have already received feedback from his teachers that his performance in school is poor. You are trying your best to tutor him at home, but to no avail. You cannot afford to hire a personal tutor for Joseph. In addition, you noticed that over the past month, there were many nights on which Joseph has been wetting the bed. You are very concerned about this and have decided to seek help from your local GP. Your local GP feels that there might be an underlying mental health issue and hence has referred you to see the child psychiatrist.

CASC Construct Table:

The CASC Construct Table is formatted so that candidates can adequately cover the range and depth of the assessment required in this station.

DOI: 10.1201/9781003313113-63

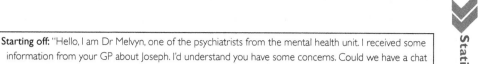

Starting off: "Hello, I am Dr Melvyn, one of the psychiatrists from the mental health unit. I received some information from your GP about Joseph. I'd understand you have some concerns. Could we have a chat about it?"			
History of the current presenting problem	Could you tell me more about your concerns? Thanks for sharing with me. I understand that it must have been difficult for you as a parent. I will be asking you lots of questions, including questions about your child's voiding pattern, his bowel function (frequency of passing a stool), and how these problems affect him.	Could you tell me roughly when you first noticed that Joseph has been wetting his bed? How has this problem progressed over the past month or so?	How often has Joseph been wetting his bed in the past week or so?
Clarifying the history of enuresis	With regard to your current concern, can I check with you whether this is the first time such a problem has occurred? Has he have had similar issues in the past? Has he been having this problem since young? Has he been dry before? How much water does he usually take before bedtime? Is there anyone in the family who has similar issues?	So it seemed like it has just started over the past month and has been progressively increasing in frequency. Is he able to stay dry in the day? Have you received any feedback from his teachers regarding this?	Does Joseph have other problems, such as him having difficulties with bowel movements? How often does he have a bowel movement? What do you do if you find out that Joseph has wet the bed? How do you usually react? How does he feel about you finding out? What does he say?
Identification of stressors	Do you have other worries for Joseph? Could you tell me more?	Apart from the concern about schoolwork and his poor performance in school, is there anything else you think might be bothering Joseph?	How have things been at home? Have there been any recent changes in the home environment? How is his relationship with yourself and the rest of the family?
Identification of other comorbid psychiatric conditions	Over the past two weeks or so, how do you think Joseph's mood has been? Is he still able to keep up with things that he used to enjoy? Does he seem to be more anxious than usual?	How has his sleep been? How has his appetite been?	Are there problems with him going to school? Does he refuse to go to school? Has a psychiatrist seen Joseph before? Has he been diagnosed with any psychiatric condition, such as ADHD?

(Continued)

(Continued)

Developmental history	Could you tell me more about his development? Was the pregnancy normal? Was the delivery normal?	Were there any issues in the early years? Did the doctors pick up any developmental delays?	Have you noted that he used to achieve his milestones much slower than the other children? Were there any previous issues with potty training?
Rule out medical comorbidity	I understand that the GP has seen him prior to referring him to our service. Do you know if blood tests as well as urine analysis were done?	Does Joseph have any underlying chronic medical conditions that I need to know of? (If he does have) Can I know the medication that he is on now? Have there been any changes to his medication recently?	Has Joseph been complaining of any difficulties with urination? Have you noticed that he needs to go to the toilet frequently? Does his urine smell foul? (If there is an underlying history of seizure) Can I know when he has had his last fit? What kind of fits does he usually have? Does he lose consciousness?

Common pitfalls:

a. Failure to cover the range and depth of the station (there is a need to take a developmental history and exclude other possible medical comorbid in this station).

b. Regarding the presenting issues of enuresis, candidates need to ask the following key questions: Is it nocturnal or diurnal? Is it primary (never been dry before) or secondary? Any associated encopresis? How much does he drink before bedtime? How do the caregivers react? Is there any family history?

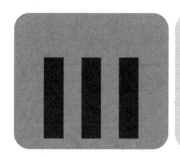

STATION 64
ELECTIVE MUTISM

Information to candidates:

Name of patient: Shane Parker

The local GP has referred Shane Parker to your service for further assessment. She has just started school in the past month, and the teachers have reported that she has refused to speak. She is noted to be totally mute and does not answer anyone in school. This behaviour of Shane is strange as she can communicate without any issues at home. You have assessed Shane, and she is also reluctant to speak to you. Her mother, Mrs Parker, is here and hopes to find out more from you.

Task: Please speak to Mrs Parker and obtain further information about her child's behaviour. Please explain your current assessment and your management approach. Finally, please address all her concerns and expectations.

Outline of station:

You are Mrs Parker, the mother of Shane. You have received feedback from the teachers informing you that Shane has been totally mute at school. You are quite surprised by this, as she can communicate normally at home. You have asked her why she is mute at school, but she becomes teary and refuses to say anything. You are quite concerned as to whether there is anything wrong with her. You have sought help from your GP, who has recommended that she see a child psychiatrist. You understand from the assessment conducted by the child psychiatrist that she was mute throughout the interview as well. You are anxious and wish to understand what is wrong with your child and how the psychiatrist could help you with her sudden behavioural change.

CASC Construct Table:

The CASC Construct Table is formatted so that candidates can adequately cover the range and depth of the assessment required in this station.

DOI: 10.1201/9781003313113-64

Starting off: "Hello, I am Dr Melvyn, one of the psychiatrists from the mental health unit. I received some information from your GP about Shane and have assessed her. I understand you have some concerns. Could we have a chat about it?"			
Assessment of selective mutism	Thanks for sharing your concerns with me. I would be asking you several questions to understand the problem better. Has there been any feedback from the teachers in school? Is she able to talk to her friends/peers in school? Does she only speak to selected friends in school? Is she able to answer questions that the teacher asks? Is she able to speak to her teacher? Is she able to speak and interact with others in a group setting?	(At home) Can you tell me more about her behaviours at home? Is she able to speak to you/her siblings? Is she able to speak to family members when there are other people present? Can she speak to family members who do not live with you?	
Explain the assessment and information needed	The information you shared with me is essential in helping us formulate the diagnosis.	In addition to the information you have provided, we might also need additional information from your GP and the school. Would that be fine with you? At times, we also request a formal school report. Is that fine with you?	Do you know if any educational psychologist has seen Shane in the school? If an educational psychologist has done so, we like to obtain some information from her regarding her assessment of Shane. In addition, I'd like to find out whether there have been any other problems at school. Do you know whether she has been bullied at school? How have things been at home? Have there been any changes in the home environment? How does she communicate at home?

Obtain developmental history	I have seen Shane in my clinic previously, but she is not willing to share much as well. I hope you can share with me more about her development in her younger years to help me understand Shane better.	Could I ask whether there were any problems whilst you had Shane? Were there any problems with the delivery and thereafter?	Could I check whether Shane met all her developmental milestones? Did any doctor inform you that Shane was developing slower than normal children? Did Shane ever have any serious childhood infection that required prolonged hospitalization? Does Shane have any chronic medical issues that I need to know of? Is she on any chronic medication?
Discuss the possible differential diagnosis	Once we have gathered more information from the school and considered the information you shared with us, we will have a better idea of the likely underlying condition causing this.	For now, it seems that what Shane is having is what is known as elective mutism. Have you heard of this before? In this condition, children tend to have issues in speaking in certain social situations.	The other conditions I like to consider might be that of emotional disorders and natural shyness.
Explain investigations	We like to suggest further investigations to determine the exact cause of the condition. As a baseline, we need to conduct a physical and neurological examination.	Psychometric testing must be beneficial. As the problems are confined to the school environment, assessment by an educational psychologist will be essential. We'd like to suggest conducting a school visit to observe her interaction in the school setting.	We will also consider referring her for further speech and language assessment to determine if she has underlying speech or language problems accounting for her not speaking in school.
Explain treatment	The modality of treatment depends on the exact cause of her problems. If she is selectively not speaking only in the school setting, we might need the psychologist to make use of behavioural methods to address this issue. In behavioural therapy, positive behaviours such as talking are rewarded in the school setting, reinforcing the positive behaviour.	If there were underlying speech or hearing abnormalities, appropriate interventions, such as speech therapy, could be conducted.	

(Continued)

(Continued)

Explain prognosis	The prognosis for the condition is usually good.		

Common pitfall:

a. Failure to assess elective mutism and ask specific questions in depth.

TOPIC IV
LEARNING DISABILITIES

STATION 65
LEARNING DISABILITY WITH CHALLENGING BEHAVIOUR (HISTORY TAKING)

Information to candidates:

Name of patient: Mr Davis

Mr Davis has a severe learning disability and has been staying in a residential home for the past two years. The home manager, Mr Thomas, called the outpatient clinic urgently, requesting an earlier appointment to see the learning disability service psychiatrist. In view of the urgency of the referral, an appointment was made to see you. Mr Thomas mentioned during the clinic consultation that Mr Davis seemed like a changed person for the past two weeks. His nursing staff in the home are finding it tremendously tough to cope with his challenging behaviours. Mr Thomas hopes you could help him with his current situation as he has not noted Mr Davis's abnormal behaviours since he has been with them.

Task: Please speak to Mr Thomas to get more history and to identify a likely cause for the changes in behaviour. Please use the available time to explain to Mr Thomas the most likely reasons for the drastic changes in behaviour.

Outline of station:

You are Mr Thomas, the manager of the home. Mr Davis has been your resident in the home for the past two years. Your staffs have noticed a dramatic change in Mr Davis's behaviour over the past two weeks. At times Mr Davis would seem to be very irritable in his mood, and at times he would refuse his meals as well as his medication. He has been refusing to participate in the usual activities he used to enjoy. Your staffs have been finding it a struggle to help Mr Davis with his behaviour and have related this to you. You are at your wit's end, so you need to arrange an earlier appointment with the psychiatrist, hoping that some medication would help fix the problem. You do know that Mr Davis has a history of seizures and has seen the neurologist recently and continued the same dose of the medication for his seizures. He has been complaining recently of pain during urination. Otherwise, there have not been other complaints. There have not been any other changes to the schedule of activities at the nursing home.

CASC Construct Table:

The CASC Construct Table is formatted such that candidates would be able adequately to cover both the range and depth of the assessment required in this station.

DOI: 10.1201/9781003313113-65

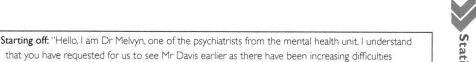

Starting off: "Hello, I am Dr Melvyn, one of the psychiatrists from the mental health unit. I understand that you have requested for us to see Mr Davis earlier as there have been increasing difficulties managing him in the nursing home. Could you tell me more about this?"			
Clarification of the history of presenting symptoms	I'm sorry to hear that it has been a difficult and challenging time for yourself and your staff. I'd like to try to understand the situation better so that we could help Mr Davis.	Could you tell me, when did these all begin? How was Mr Davis before these all began? Could you tell me more about his difficult behaviours? What did he do? Are there times to which he is aggressive?	When Mr Davis has those challenging behaviours, how did your nurses handle him? Does he require any additional doses of medication to calm him down? Has something like this happened before in the past?
Consider and exclude mood disorders and psychosis	Could you tell me how David's mood has been? Does he seem to be very irritable or tearful at times? Is he still able to enjoy things he used to enjoy doing? Has he been refusing to participate in leisure activities or work? Is he still performing in his work?	How has his sleep been? How has his appetite been? Is he able to handle his own personal care?	Are there times to which he seems preoccupied? Are there times when he seems to be responding to voices or external stimuli? How has he been getting on with the rest of the residents in the home?
Consider and exclude medical disorders	Could you tell me whether he has other underlying medical conditions that I need to know of? (Or) Is he on any long-term medication that I need to know of? Have there been any recent changes in his medication?	Has he taken ill recently? Could you tell me more about his recent illness? Did he seek any medical help for his recent illness?	
Consider and exclude changes in the environment	Could you share with me whether there have been any changes in your home environment?	Have there been any new nursing staff in your home? Have there been any new residents in the home?	Do you know whether Mr Davis's parents have visited him recently? Have they provided any inputs about his behaviour?

(Continued)

(Continued)

| Psychoeducation about reasons for behavioural change | Thanks for sharing your concerns with me. I have a better understanding of the problem.
It seems to me that there might be a variety of reasons as to why Mr Davis has had a change in behaviour. | I am concerned that there have been some changes in the environment that he is placed in. In addition, I am concerned that there are changes in the doses of the medication that he has been using for his epilepsy condition. | I need to discuss Mr Davis's case with my consultant to see how best we could help you. Do you have any other questions for me? |

Common pitfalls:

   a. Failure to explore the possibility of other physical conditions causing the changes in behaviour.

   b. Failure to explore the possibility of changes in the environment resulting in behavioural changes.

   c. Failure to elicit specific features associated with depression in people with learning disabilities (e.g. tantrums, challenging behaviours, low self-esteem).

It is important to note that the clinical features of depression in adults with learning disabilities tend to vary with the level of disability; in those with higher levels of disability, irritability and anger, self-injurious and aggressive behaviour, psychomotor changes, and loss of activities of daily living skills may be observed rather than the classic depressive symptoms. (Davis JP, Judd FK, Herrman H. Depression in adults with intellectual disability. Part 1: A review. Aust N Z J Psychiatry. 1997 Apr;31(2):232–42. doi: 10.3109/00048679709073826. PMID: 9140631.)

Information to candidates:

Name of patient: Mr Mohri

The local GP has referred Joseph Mohri to the learning disability service. His brother, Thomas, has previously brought him for an assessment with their local GP as Thomas has been very concerned about Joseph's declining memory and his need for more assistance in his daily activities. Joseph has been previously diagnosed with mild learning disability and has been able to work previously in a sheltered workshop up till one year ago.

Task: Please speak to Thomas Mohri, Joseph's brother, to obtain further history to arrive at a diagnosis. Please also perform an appropriate risk assessment based on the history and the diagnosis you are suspecting.

Outline of station:

You are Mr Thomas Mohri, the brother of Joseph. Joseph has been diagnosed with mild learning disability since the age of 8 years. He is capable of independent living and previously managed to sustain a job at the local handicraft workshop until last year. He was dismissed from his job due to his poor work performance. Over the past year, you have been noticing that Joseph is no longer his usual self. He has been having progressive difficulties with his short-term memories. However, his long-term memory is still intact. At times, he does seem to be confused about the day and the dates as well. He is having more difficulty finding the right words to say at the right time. He also requires more assistance in terms of daily living, especially in finances. You are also particularly concerned about the risks involved when he is alone at home. There was an occasion to which he forgot to switch off the gas. You are hoping that, by speaking to the psychiatrist today, you could know what is going wrong for Joseph.

CASC Construct Table:

The CASC Construct Table is formatted so that candidates can adequately cover the range and depth of the assessment required in this station.

DOI: 10.1201/9781003313113-66

Starting off: "Hello, I am Dr Melvyn, one of the psychiatrists from the mental health unit. I understand that the GP has referred your brother to see us early as you have some concerns. Could we have a chat about it?"

Clarification about the presenting complaint	I understand that you have brought your brother to see the GP because of your concerns about his memory difficulties. Could you tell me more?	Could you tell me, when did these memory difficulties first start? (Or) How long has there been difficulties with his memory?	How have things been recently? I'm sorry to hear that things have been worsening. It must have been a very difficult time for you.
Exploration of memory difficulties	Have there been any problems with his short-term memory? By that, I mean, are there times to which he misplaces things? Have there been times to which he forgets his meal?	What about his memories for things in the past? Could he still remember things that have happened years ago?	Would you say that his memory is progressively getting worse since the time to which it first started?
Exploration of orientation and visuospatial dysfunction	Does he seem to get muddled up with the day and the dates in a week?	Have there been times to which you noticed that he seemed to be very confused?	Is he able to recognize loved ones? What about distant relatives that he hardly meets?
Exploration of language, communication, and recognition difficulties	Have there been times when he has difficulties finding the right words in a conversation?	Are there times when he seemed to have great difficulties understanding a normal conversation?	Is he able to recognize and identify everyday objects? Can he find the right words to name those objects?
Exploration of functioning	Is he still able to manage himself? Could you tell me more about the difficulties that he has been having?	Does he require additional help with any of the following? – Finances – Shopping – Food preparation – Transportation	Does he need additional help with any of the following? – Dressing – Washing – Toileting – Ambulation
Assessment of other psychiatric disorders	How has his mood been recently? Is he still able to enjoy the things that he used to enjoy previously?	How has his sleep been? How has his appetite been?	Have you noticed whether he has any abnormal behaviours?
Risk assessment	Have there been any other concerns with regard to his behaviour of late?	Has he been aggressive verbally or physically at home? Has he accidentally hurt himself recently?	Has he wandered out of the house previously? Has he done anything dangerous at home recently? Thanks for sharing your concerns with me.

Common pitfalls:

a. Failure to cover the range and depth of the information necessary to make a diagnosis of dementia.
b. Failure to cover a comprehensive risk assessment.

Information to candidates:

Name of patient: Mr Dewitt

The local GP has referred Mr Dewitt, a gentleman previously diagnosed with a mild learning disability, to your specialist outpatient service. His family members have noticed that, over the past month, he has been increasingly withdrawn and low in mood.

Task: Please speak to Mr Dewitt and elicit features of depression. Please also perform an appropriate risk assessment.

Outline of station:

You are Mr Dewitt, and you have been asked to come to see the psychiatrist by your family. Over the past month, you have been having low mood. You used to be able to work in the nearby store owned by your family doing simple chores, but, over the past month, you have found yourself having no energy for work at all. You find it tough to go to sleep at night and you do not have much appetite as well. You have also lost a significant amount of weight over the past month. You do not have any suicidal ideations.

CASC Construct Table:

The CASC Construct Table is formatted so that candidates can adequately cover the range and depth of the assessment required in this station.

Starting off: "Hello, I am Dr Melvyn, one of the psychiatrists from the mental health unit. I understand that the GP has referred you to see us today. Could we have a chat?"			
History of presenting complaint	I understand that you have been having some difficulties lately. Could you please tell me more?	I'm sorry to hear about all this. How long have you been troubled by these difficulties?	(Or) Do you know when all these difficulties first started? Do you feel that things are worsening?

DOI: 10.1201/9781003313113-67

Core clinical features of depression	How has your mood been recently?	You mentioned that your mood has not been good. Have you been more emotional and been crying more recently? If I were to ask you to rate your mood on a scale from 1 to 10, where 1 is low and 10 is happy, what number would you give your mood?	What are your hobbies? Have you still been able to enjoy things you used to enjoy? Do you find that you have lost interest in things you previously liked to do?
Biological symptoms of depression	How has your energy been? Do you feel you don't have the energy to do everything?	How has your sleep been? Do you wake up earlier in the morning?	How has your appetite been? Do you find that you have lost a lot of weight recently?
Other depressive features	Could you watch a television programme?	How confident do you feel in yourself? Do you feel that you're as good as others?	Do you feel that you have done something wrong? Do you blame yourself for anything? I understand that this has been a very stressful time for you. Have you had any unusual experiences when stressed? Such as hearing voices?
Risk assessment	Do you feel that life is no longer worth living? Do you feel that you are better off dead?	Have you had thoughts of ending your life? Have you made any plans?	Thanks for sharing and for speaking to me.

Common pitfalls:

a. Failure to communicate effectively and to tailor questions in accordance with the intelligence level of the individual.

b. Failure to elicit specific features associated with depression in people with learning disabilities.

Information to candidates:

Name of patient: Mr Porter

The local GP has referred Mr Emerson Porter to the emergency department. In the memo, it is stated that Mr Porter is a 25-year-old male with a history of mild learning disability. He has been recently seen by a psychiatrist and has been started on an antidepressant known as dothiepin for his sleep and for his mood symptoms. Since the commencement of the antidepressant, it was stated that his family have noted that Johnson does behave out of the norm at times. There were times during a conversation to when he lost consciousness. This has never happened before. The GP is concerned and hence has referred him urgently to the emergency services for further evaluation. Mr Porter is here with you in the emergency, with his elder brother, Thompson.

Task: Please speak to his elder brother, Mr Thompson Porter, to understand more about what has been happening. Please elicit more information to arrive at a possible diagnosis.

Outline of station:

You are Mr Thompson Porter, the brother of Emerson. Over the last month, you have noticed on multiple occasions that your brother does not seem the same as before. You know that your brother has seen a psychiatrist one month ago and have been started on an antidepressant for his sleep and mood symptoms. Over the course of the last month, you noticed that he blanks out at times during a normal conversation. At times, before these episodes, he would report experiencing visual disturbances and hallucinations. During those episodes, he would initially still be partially aware of his surroundings, but it would progress to him being dazed and being unresponsive to commands. During those episodes, he has been observed lip smacking and motor movements. Thereafter, he usually complains of feeling confused and sleepy. You are very concerned about the reasons accounting for this change in behaviour. Your brother does not have any other medical history of note, but there is a family history of seizures within the family.

CASC Construct Table:

The CASC Construct Table is formatted so that candidates can adequately cover the range and depth of the assessment required in this station.

DOI: 10.1201/9781003313113-68

Starting off: "Hello, I am Dr Melvyn, one of the psychiatrists from the mental health unit. I understand that the GP has referred your brother to see us today. Could we have a chat for us to understand more about his condition?"

Presenting complaint	I understand how difficult it must have been for you given your worries for your brother. I hope to understand more from you to better help your brother with his condition.	Could you tell me the changes that you have noticed? When did this first begin? Or how long has there been these changes in behaviour?	How frequently have you been noticing such changes? Have these changes in behaviour been progressively worsening?
Pre-ictal	Could you tell me what usually happens before your brother has an episode of this abnormal behaviour? Does he describe experiencing any unusual experiences or feelings?	Does he seem to stare blankly into space?	Does he seem to be totally unresponsive to external commands? Are there any abnormal involuntary movements that you have observed prior to the onset of those episodes? Does he have any abnormal movements in his mouth or limbs?
Ictal phase	Could you tell me what happens then? Do you know roughly how long these episodes last?	Does he lose total consciousness during those episodes? Or does he seem to be still aware of his surroundings?	Besides losing consciousness, does he have other abnormal movements during those episodes? Has he ever lost continence during those episodes?
Post-ictal phase	Could you tell me more about what happens after each episode?	Does he appear to be confused or sleepy?	Does he remember what happened during the episode itself? Does he complain of any headache?
Medical history	I understand that your brother has a history of learning disability and has just been in recent contact with his psychiatrist. Do you know whether he has been on chronic medication from the psychiatrist? Have there been any recent changes in his medication that you are aware of?	Does your brother have any underlying medical conditions that I need to know of? Is he on any other chronic medication? Does he use any other substances such as alcohol or any other drugs?	Can I check whether there is a family history of seizures? Thanks for sharing with me this information.

Common pitfalls:

a. Failure to cover the range and depth of the information required for this station.

b. Failure to ask questions that assess specifically for temporal lobe epilepsy.

Information to candidates:

Name of patient: Mr Legrand

Dorothy is the mother of Mr John Legrand, a 30-year-old male who has been previously diagnosed with mild learning disability. He has been staying at a residential home because Dorothy, his mother, needs to work long hours to make ends meet. Recently, Dorothy has learnt that John has had a relationship with another female member at the residential home, and the girl is currently four months pregnant. Dorothy has requested for an early appointment to see you as she has quite a few concerns.

Task: Please speak to Dorothy, the mother of John Legrand, and address all her concerns and expectations.

Outline of station:

You are Dorothy, the mother of John Legrand. John has been diagnosed with mild learning disability since young. You had a hard time raising him, coupled with the fact that your husband has left home as he could not accept the fact that John has a learning disability. You learnt about John having a girlfriend only two months back. You are now very surprised to know that the girl is four months pregnant. You are very concerned that in view of John and his girlfriend's intellectual disabilities, the child would be removed from them by social services. In addition, you are also doubtful whether they could parent the child. You are very worried that you might end up being the one who is supposed to parent the child. You are also very worried that your grandchild might have a learning disability. You wonder why individuals with learning disabilities are not sterilized. You appeared extremely distressed throughout the interview.

CASC Construct Table:

The CASC Construct Table is formatted such that candidates would be able to cover adequately both the range and depth of the assessment required in this station.

DOI: 10.1201/9781003313113-69

Starting off: "Hello, I am Dr Melvyn, one of the psychiatrists from the mental health unit. I understand that you have some concerns about John, your son. Could we have a chat about it?"			
History of presenting complaint	I have some understanding of what has happened. Could you share with me more about what your concerns are?	I understand how difficult it must have been for you. Thanks for sharing with me.	Do you know when your son first met his current girlfriend? Do you know roughly how many months into a pregnancy his girlfriend is into?
Parenting of child	I understand that John has underlying mild learning disabilities. Do you recall when it was first diagnosed? Did the doctors tell he had learning disabilities? How has he been coping ever since? Is he able to do things independently? Or does he need assistance even for very simple daily tasks? Is he currently working? If so, how is his work performance? Do you know more about John's girlfriend? Do you know what extent of learning disabilities she has? Are you aware of how independent she is? Does she require assistance even in daily activities?	I hear that you have some concerns about the social services taking away your grandchild. Am I right in saying so? My understanding is that the social workers would not automatically take away the child. Usually, when the child is born, they will conduct a series of parenting assessments to determine whether your son and his girlfriend can take care of the child. There are also several programmes that your son and his girlfriend can attend during the pregnancy, to help them prepare for taking care of the baby. After birth, social services can provide further training.	Very often, only in exceptional cases to which both parents do not have the capacity would the child be taken away for alternative care arrangements. I understand your concerns about them imposing upon you to take care of your grandson. I'm sorry to hear how difficult it was previously when you had John. Let me reassure you that the social work would make the best arrangement in this circumstance.
Sterilization	Thanks for bringing up this issue regarding sterilization for John and his girlfriend.	Even though John and his girlfriend have mild learning disabilities, it does not necessarily mean that they cannot have children. They do have the same rights as any other human being. Moreover, sterilization is a surgical procedure and requires the consent of your son and his girlfriend.	Only in exceptional circumstances, when there is a lack of capacity for both individuals, would a court be involved. The decision would have to be in the best medical interest for your son.

(Continued)

(Continued)

| Possibility of child having learning disabilities | I hear your concerns about your grandchild having learning disabilities as well. Before I address that, could I check with you how John was diagnosed with learning disability? Is there anyone in the family with a history of learning disability, apart from John? | There are a variety of causes for learning disabilities. Inheritance plays a role, but there are also many other factors in place. | Are you aware whether his girlfriend has gone for any antenatal checks? The underlying reason this needs to be done is to facilitate early pickup of abnormalities. |

Common pitfall:

a. Failure to cover the range and depth of the information required for this station.

Information to candidates:

Name of patient: Mr Flint

You have been tasked to speak to the key worker for Mr Charlie Flint, a 25-year-old male who has a history of moderate learning disability. The key worker has requested for an earlier consultation as he is concerned that Charlie has been increasingly withdrawn in the day centre. However, he used to have interest and was still able to participate in the daily activities in the day centre up till two weeks ago.

Task: Please speak to Mr Flint's key worker to assess for the potential causes leading to his current presentation. Please obtain enough information to come to a diagnosis.

Outline of station:

You are the key worker of Mr Charlie Flint. You are very concerned about the acute behavioural changes that you have noted over the past two weeks. You noticed that Mr Flint has been increasingly withdrawn over the past two weeks. This took place immediately after he went back home during the weekend with his parents. When he returned, you have noticed some bruising over his bilateral arms. Charlie is not able to tell you the reasons as to why he has the bruises. You have contacted his parents to find out more information, to which they have claimed he might have hurt himself accidentally. Charlie does have an underlying medical condition (that of epilepsy), but he has not had a seizure for the past year. Owing to his degree of learning disability, he is only able to gesture to indicate his needs. Over the past two weeks, he has been more withdrawn and does not even gesture to indicate his needs.

CASC Construct Table:

The CASC Construct Table is formatted such that candidates would be able to cover adequately both the range and depth of the assessment required in this station.

DOI: 10.1201/9781003313113-70

Starting off: "Hello, I am Dr Melvyn, one of the psychiatrists from the mental health unit. I understand that you have some concerns about Charlie Flint, one of your residents in your home. Could we have a chat about it?"		
History of presenting complaint	I understand that you have some concerns about how Charlie has been. Could you tell me more about it?	I'm sorry to learn that. Could you please kindly let me know when this first started. (Or) How long has Charlie had these changes in behaviour?	Do you feel that the changes in behaviour are progressively worsening? (Or) Have there been further changes in his behaviour since you first noticed it?
Exploration of social circumstances	You mentioned that the changes first started after the outing that Charlie has had with his parents. Could you share with me more about his relationship with his family? How often is he allowed to head home and spend time with his family? Does his family visit him at the home he is currently living in?	You mentioned that you have noticed some bruises the last time Charlie came back from home leave. Have you asked him about it? Have you asked his parents about the bruises?	Has there been any of the following concerns previously? (Psychological/emotional abuse) For example, do his parents call him names and put him down? (Financial abuse) Have there been concerns as to whether he has been provided with adequate finances? (Neglect) Have there been other concerns about neglect when he is back on home leave?
Exploration of comorbid psychiatric symptoms	I am concerned to hear that Charlie has been more withdrawn recently. Could you tell me more? Does it mean to say that Charlie is no longer able to enjoy activities he used to enjoy?	How has his mood been recently over the past two weeks? Have your workers in the home noticed any change in his sleep? Does Charlie seem to be having poor appetite?	Apart from being withdrawn, are there any other abnormal behaviours that your staffs have noticed? Is he more aggressive and violent in the residential home? Also, does he seem more easily startled recently?
Establishment of baseline communication and skills	For me to understand the problem better, I'd like to understand more about how Charlie was like before all these happened. My understanding is that Charlie has moderate learning disability. Am I right?	Could you tell me how Charlie usually communicates his needs? Is he able to say any words? Does he use only gestures? What activities of daily living could Charlie perform independently?	How does Charlie interact with the rest of the residents of the home? Does Charlie have any issues with any of the residents?

| Exclude medical causes | Can I check whether Charlie has any underlying medical conditions that I need to know of? If so, is he on long-term chronic medication? | You mentioned that he does have epilepsy. Do you know when was the last time he had a fit? Has his medication for his epilepsy been adjusted recently? | Thanks for sharing with me. Do you have other concerns you wish to share? |

Common pitfalls:

a. Failure to cover the range and depth of the information required for this station.
b. Superficial assessment of abuse and lack of depth.

TOPIC V
ADDICTIONS AND SUBSTANCE MISUSE

STATION 71
ALCOHOL
DEPENDENCE (HISTORY
TAKING)

Information to candidates:

Name of patient: Mr Samuels

The local GP has referred Mr Samuels to your service. His recent blood tests done with the local GP has shown that he has a deranged liver function test. His local GP has written you a memo asking you to help evaluate his condition as he understands that Mr Samuels has been a chronic drinker for years.

Task: Please speak to Mr Samuels and elicit a history to diagnose alcohol dependence.

Outline of station:

You are Mr Samuels, and your local GP has referred you to see the psychiatrist. You are ambivalent about attending today's appointment, but you are quite concerned about learning recently that your liver is not working fine. Your local GP has told you that it might be due to the alcohol you have used over the years. You started drinking when you were a teenager and previously used only beer. Recently, due to stressors from work and from your relationships, you have been using more alcohol to cope. You are beginning to find that you need more to get the same effect, and you need to drink to avoid getting bad withdrawals. You are here to see if the psychiatrist could provide additional help to help you with this drinking problem.

CASC Construct Table:

The CASC Construct Table is formatted such that candidates would be able to cover adequately both the range and depth of the assessment required in this station.

Starting off: "Hello, I am Dr Melvyn, one of the psychiatrists from the mental health unit. I understand that your GP has referred you to our service, as he has shared some concerns about your recent liver function test. Could we have a chat?"			
History of presenting complaint	Could I understand more about you and what your GP has told you? Did he inform you of the possible reasons for the changes in your blood test?	Could you share with me more about your usual drinking habits? Could you tell me when you first started to drink? What did you start drinking?	How have things changed since the time you first started drinking? Could you take me through a typical day and tell me more about your drinking patterns?

(Continued)

(Continued)

Compulsive drinking, tolerance, and withdrawals	Do you sometimes find it difficult to control the amount of alcohol you use? How long have you been feeling this way for?	Do you find that you need to drink much more to feel the similar effects from alcohol you have consumed?	Have you missed a drink before? What would happen if you missed a drink? Do you get bad tremors if you do not drink? Have there been any episodes to which you were confused and do not know your whereabouts? When was the last time this happened? Were there times to which you missed your drink and have had unusual experiences?
Primacy, relief drinking, reinstatement, stereotype	Would you say that alcohol has been a priority for you? Is it far more important to get a drink than other commitments you have in life?	Do you start drinking the first thing in the morning? With whom do you usually drink together with?	Have you tried to stop drinking previously? What happens when you attempt to stop drinking?
Complications	How has your alcohol problem affected you? How has it affected your physical health? Blackouts, fits, gastric, liver dysfunction, memory impairment, sexual dysfunction, etc.	Apart from it affecting your physical health, has it affected your work?	Has your drinking problem affected your relationships? Have you got into any trouble with the law because of your drinking habits?
Current mental state	I understand that you are concerned about your health and drinking habits. Can I check how your mood has been recently? What about your interest? Are you able to enjoy the things you used to enjoy previously?	How has your sleep been recently? What about your appetite?	Have there been times in which you experienced hearing voices, even when you are sober? Have there been any difficulties in your relationships? (Screen for morbid jealousy) Do you feel in control of your actions and emotions? Have you recently felt that life is not worth living or is meaningless?
Insight and readiness for change	Do you feel that you might have a problem with alcohol? What makes you feel so?	How do you want us to help you with your alcohol problem?	Do you have any questions for me?

Common pitfalls:

a. Failure to cover the range and depth of the information required for this station.
b. Failure to assess the complications that might have arisen from his current drinking habits.
c. Failure to assess for insight and readiness for change.

It is important to be familiar with Prochaska and DiClement's stages of change.

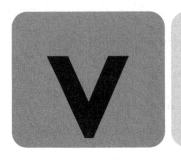

Information to candidates:

Name of patient: Mr Samuels

The patient, who has been previously assessed, has been admitted to the medical ward as he sustained a fall whilst he was out drinking. The medical team has completed their work-up for his condition, but they are hoping that the psychiatrist could review him before he is allowed home. His wife, Sarah, is here and wants to find out more about his condition.

Task: Please speak to Mrs Sarah Samuels, his wife, and address all her concerns and expectations.

Outline of station:

You are Sarah, the wife of Mr Samuels. You are aware that he has been admitted to the hospital following a fall whilst he was intoxicated last night. You are very worried about the complications of his long-term alcohol dependence. You wish to know more about how best the addiction team here could help him with his condition. You wish to know whether there are medications and talking therapies that might be effective for him.

CASC Construct Table:

The CASC Construct Table is formatted such that candidates would be able to cover adequately both the range and depth of the assessment required in this station.

Starting off: "Hello, I am Dr Melvyn, one of the psychiatrists from the mental health unit. I understand that you have some concerns about your husband, Mr Samuels. Could we have a chat about this?"			
Updates about the current condition	I'm sorry to inform you that your husband was admitted to the medical ward following a fall whilst intoxicated.	Since the time that he has been admitted, our medical team has worked him up, and he is stable now. I'd like to reassure you that they have called me to speak to your husband and yourself as we understand you have some concerns about his condition.	Could you share with me more about your concerns? Could you share with me how long you have realized that your husband has had a problem with alcohol?

DOI: 10.1201/9781003313113-72

Explanation of the complications associated with alcohol dependence	Thanks for sharing your concerns. I understand that it must have been a very difficult time for you. Are you aware of the complications that might arise from long-term alcohol usage?	Several complications might arise because of long-term alcohol usage. It might cause physical health problems. Alcohol is acted upon by the liver, and very often the liver might be affected. The acute withdrawal of alcohol might also precipitate seizures or fits in some individuals.	In addition, patients with chronic alcohol dependence are also at risk towards the development of other comorbid psychiatric conditions, such as depression and anxiety. Sometimes, patients with chronic alcoholism might also get into trouble with the law (such as due to drunk driving). In the long run, there is a concern that the chronic usage of alcohol might induce what is commonly known as alcoholic dementia.
Management approach	Thanks for coming down today. I hope to discuss with you several options we could adopt to help your husband with this condition. Your continued support would determine the success of the treatment programme.	There are programmes such as alcohol detoxification programmes that your husband might benefit from.	I would like to discuss with you some medications, therapies, and other help that I feel might benefit your husband. Is it all right for me to move on to share this information with you?
Pharmacology management	In terms of medication, there are several options. If your husband is agreeable for a detoxification programme, we will start him on a tapering dose of hypnotics to help him with the withdrawal symptoms.	Other medications have been licensed for use. There are anti-craving medications, such as naltrexone. Naltrexone is usually started upon the completion of one's detoxification treatment.	Naltrexone works by binding to the opioid receptors in the body and blocking the effects and feelings of alcohol. This medication helps to reduce cravings and the amount consumed. In addition to naltrexone, there are also medications that would help him to maintain abstinence, such as acamprosate. This medication also acts on the central nervous system and helps maintain abstinence in alcohol-dependent individuals.

(Continued)

(Continued)

Psychological management	Apart from medication, there are other forms of therapy that might benefit him.	We could refer him to a psychologist for talking therapy such as cognitive behavioural therapy.	At times, brief interventions such as FRAMES (feedback, responsibility, advice, menu of strategies, empathy, and self-efficacy) could also be utilized to help patients with their symptoms.
Social management	We need your continued help to help your husband be abstinent from alcohol.	In addition, we could link him up with support groups such as Alcoholic Anonymous.	
Prognosis	The good prognostic factors for the condition include having an insight into the condition.	In addition, a close network of support from family and friends also promises a better prognosis.	I understand that I have shared quite a lot of information today. Could I leave you with some leaflets about what we have discussed today?

Common pitfalls:

a. Failure to cover the range and depth of the information required for this station.
b. Failure to discuss alternative medication apart from recommending a detoxification programme.
c. Failure to discuss social factors such as family and GP support.

STATION 73
EFFECTS OF ALCOHOL ON MOOD (HISTORY TAKING)

Information to candidates:

Name of patient: Mr Rogers

Mr Rogers has been referred by his local GP to your service. You note that the referral memo states that the patient has a long-standing history of alcohol consumption. He has been referred to your service today as the patient has been having one month's worth of low mood with fleeting suicidal ideations.

Task: Please speak to Mr Rogers and obtain a brief history of his drinking habits and the impact of his habits on his mood.

Outline of station:

You are Mr Rogers. You have visited your GP as you have been feeling low for the past month, with a reduction in interest in doing things you used to enjoy. Your work performance has deteriorated, and there have been relationship issues with your wife as well. You have difficulties with sleep, and your appetite is poor. In view of your stressors, you have been coping by increasing your alcohol intake. You thought that alcohol could help you get over this difficult period. There were several occasions to which you have had fleeting thoughts of hurting yourself, but you did not succumb to that. You are desperate for help and hope that the psychiatrist can help you.

CASC Construct Table:

The CASC Construct Table is formatted so that candidates can adequately cover the range and depth of the assessment required in this station.

Starting off: "Hello, I am Dr Melvyn, one of the psychiatrists from the mental health unit. I understand that your GP has referred you to our service. Could we have a chat?"			
History of presenting complaint	I understand from the memo from my colleague that you have been feeling low in your mood and have been using alcohol to help you cope. Before we explore more about your mood, could I get a general understanding of your drinking habits?	Could you share with me more about your usual drinking habits? Could you tell me when you first started to drink? What did you start drinking?	How have things changed since the time you first started drinking? Could you take me through a typical day and tell me more about your drinking patterns?

(Continued)

DOI: 10.1201/9781003313113-73

(Continued)

Compulsive drinking, tolerance, and withdrawals	Do you find it difficult at times to control the amount of alcohol you use? How long have you been feeling this way for? Do you find that you need to drink much more in order to feel the similar effects from alcohol you have consumed?	Have you missed a drink before? What would happen if you missed a drink? Do you get bad tremors if you do not drink?	Have there been any episodes to which you lose consciousness or went into a fit? When was the last time this happened? Were there times when you missed your drink and had unusual experiences?
Primacy, relief drinking, reinstatement, stereotype	Would you say that alcohol has been a priority for you? Is it far more important to get a drink than other commitments you have in life?	Do you start drinking the first thing in the morning? With whom do you usually drink together with?	Have you tried to stop drinking previously? What happens when you attempt to stop drinking?
Complications	How has your alcohol problem affected you?	Apart from it affecting your physical health, has it affected your work?	Has your drinking problem affected your relationships? Have you got into any trouble with the law because of your drinking habits?
Assessment of depressive symptoms	Thanks for sharing with me your drinking history and habits. I'd like to understand more about your mood. Can I check, how has your mood been recently? Does your mood vary across the day? What about your interest? Are you able to enjoy the things you used to enjoy previously?	How has your sleep been recently? What about your appetite? How has your energy levels been? Are you still able to cope up with your routine daily chores? Have you made mistakes at work recently? How do you find your attention and concentration to be like?	Sometimes, when people are under stress, they do report of having unusual experiences. Have you had any unusual experiences recently? Have you have had experiences to which you feel extremely guilty? Is your low mood related to your drinking, as it seemed like your alcohol use has affected your work and caused both relationships and financial problems?
Risk assessment	Are there times to which you find that life no longer has a meaning for you?	Have you felt that life is not worth living?	Do you have any plans to do anything to end your life?

Common pitfalls:

a. Failure to cover the range and depth of the information required for this station.

b. There are two parts to the task; hence, candidates must allocate sufficient time for both tasks.

c. Candidates are expected to ask whether the depression is due to alcohol withdrawal, work and relationship impairment, financial problems associated with alcohol use, sexual dysfunction, or concerns of physical health associated with alcohol use.

d. It is crucial to perform a risk assessment in a patient who is depressed, and this should not be neglected.

Information to candidates:

Name of patient: Mr Rogers

Mr Rogers has been referred to your addiction clinic by his GP. In the referral memo, it was stated that Mr Rogers has a long-standing history of alcohol usage. Due to his alcohol usage, he has been facing some difficulties in his relationships, work, and with the police. He is keen to seek further help.

Task: Please speak to Mr Rogers and explore his current level of alcohol consumption. Please also assess his social and legal problems associated with his current long-standing history of alcohol usage.

Outline of station:

You are Mr Rogers, and your GP has referred you to the local addiction services to get some help for your alcohol problem. You have been a chronic drinker and need to drink daily, or else you would have several withdrawal side effects. Because of your chronic drinking habits, you have gotten into fights, and the police have been involved. There was an occasion in which you were also caught for drunk driving. In addition, you are not performing well in your work, and your company has dismissed you. You are having problems with your finances. Also, things are not working out well for your relationship. You have had frequent fights with your wife, who is not agreeable with your drinking habits. You are keen to seek help.

CASC Construct Table:

The CASC Construct Table is formatted such that candidates would be able to cover adequately both the range and depth of the assessment required in this station.

Starting off: "Hello, I am Dr Melvyn, one of the psychiatrists from the mental health unit. I understand that your GP has referred you to our service. Could we have a chat?"			
Current usage of alcohol	I understand from the memo from my colleague that you have been having several problems because of your long-term drinking. Before we explore more about your problems, could I get a general understanding of your drinking habits?	Could you share with me more about your usual drinking habits? Could you tell me when you first started to drink? What did you start drinking?	How have things changed since the time you first started drinking? Could you take me through a typical day and tell me more about your drinking patterns?

DOI: 10.1201/9781003313113-74

Work-related complications	Do you have any problems with regards to work due to your current problems with drinking?	Have there been days to which you were late for work? How often has this occurred? Have you missed days at work due to your problems with drinking?	Have you been less attentive and making work mistakes due to your current drinking habits?
Relationship-related complications	Do you have any problems with regard to your relationships due to your current problems with drinking?	Have you been having arguments and fights with your partner recently? Has there been a time to which you have been aggressive towards your partner?	Have there been problems with intimacy? Do you have problems sustaining an erection after alcohol use? Have you been suspecting that your partner has been unfaithful?
Forensic complications	Have you got involved with the police due to your problems with drinking?	Have you been involved in any drunk driving offences?	Have you been drunk, and have you been involved in fights when you were drunk? Are there any outstanding charges against you now?
Financial complications	Could you tell me whether you are having financial difficulties due to your current drinking habits?	Could you tell me how you have been financing your alcohol habits?	Have you borrowed money to finance your drinking habits? Did you need to reply on any social welfare support in view of your financial difficulties?
Social complications	How has drinking affected your social life?		

Common pitfalls:

a. Failure to cover the range and depth of the information required for this station.

b. Failure to elicit specific alcohol complications, for example, erectile dysfunction that leads to mistrust in one's partner, lying, absence from work after the weekend, drunk driving, etc.

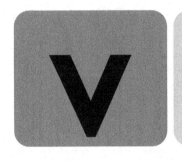

Information to candidates:

Name of patient: Mr Aronovich

You have been tasked to speak to Mr Aronovich, who has been referred to the dual addictions service by his GP. The GP has written in the memo that Mr Aronovich has a history of opioid dependence.

Task: Please speak to Mr Aronovich to elicit a history of opiate dependence.

Outline of station:

You are Mr Aronovich, and your GP has referred you to see the drug and addiction service. You were at your GP two days ago because of an infection around the site where you inject heroin. You have been using heroin since you were a teenager but have escalated over the past two years given work-related stress and relationship difficulties. You have not used any other drugs. You do use alcohol on an occasional basis. You use heroin via both the intranasal route as well as the intravenous route. You used to share needles but have not done so recently as you are aware that there is a chance you might acquire an infection such as HIV. You cannot afford to stop using heroin as you will experience significant withdrawal symptoms. You do not have any other features of any other psychiatric disorder. You feel that you need some help after the GP counselled you about the risk associated with continued usage of the drug.

CASC Construct Table:

The CASC Construct Table is formatted so that candidates can adequately cover the range and depth of the assessment required in this station.

Starting off: "Hello, I am Dr Melvyn, one of the psychiatrists from the mental health unit. I understand that your GP has referred you to our service. Could we have a chat?"			
History of presenting complaint	I understand from your GP that you have been using heroin. Could you tell me more about your usage of heroin? Apart from heroin, are there other drugs that you have been using? Do you use alcohol as well? How often and how much do you use?	Could you tell me when you first started using heroin? How much of heroin did you use when you first started? How do you use heroin? Do you "chase the dragon"?	Currently, how much of heroin do you use on a typical day? Could you take me through a typical day to help me understand your drug usage? How do you use heroin? Do you inject heroin? Have you shared needles before? How much do you spend on drugs daily?

DOI: 10.1201/9781003313113-75

Dependence symptoms	Do you feel that, recently, you needed to use more and more heroin to achieve the same effects?	Are you finding it tougher to control the amount of heroin that you are using?	Are there times when you find yourself having cravings when you miss a dose?
Withdrawal symptoms	Could you tell me more about what happens if you miss a dose or stop using heroin?	Do you experience any withdrawal symptoms? Could you tell me more about the symptoms that you have been experiencing? Have you ever had a seizure or fit if you miss a dose?	The typical withdrawal symptoms include the following: – Muscular aches – Stomach cramps – Nauseated feeling – Yawning – Rhinorrhoea Have you used any other substances, for example, cough mixture or other painkiller, to replace your heroin, should heroin not be available?
Complications	I understand that you have been using heroin intravenously. Have there been any complications from where you have been injecting? Have you had infections such as abscess? Do you have any blood-borne infections, such as hepatitis? Do you know your HIV status?	Have you ever needed to be admitted to the hospital due to the infection? Has anyone done any tests for your underlying liver condition? Do you know if you have any specific liver conditions?	How has your drug usage affected you? Has it affected your work? Has it affected your relationships? Has it affected you in terms of your finances? Have you got into trouble with the law?
Comorbid psychiatric disorders	How has your mood been recently? Do you find yourself being able to enjoy things that you used to be able to enjoy?	How have you been coping with your sleep and appetite? How is your attention and concentration?	Have you ever had any unusual experiences, such as listening to voices or seeing things that are not there? Have you ever felt that life is not worth living? Have you also been using other substances or alcohol?
Insight and motivation	Do you think you could have a mental health problem?	What do you want to do about your current problem?	What kind of help do you want from us with regards to your problem? How motivated are you for a change?

Common pitfalls:

a. Failure to cover the range and depth of the information required for this station.

b. Failure to elicit specific opioid withdrawal symptoms and complications due to intravenous use.

Information to candidates:

Name of patient: Ms Sheene

Ms Sheene is a 31-year-old female known previously to the drug and alcohol services as she has been using heroin since young. She has been maintained on methadone treatment, and she has been compliant with her methadone treatment thus far. She has missed a period for the past two months and has just discovered that she is currently pregnant. She has informed her partner about her pregnancy. Her partner is supportive and has recommended that she come by the drug and alcohol services for an evaluation as he is concerned about her continued usage of methadone whilst she is pregnant. You are the core trainee on call, and you have been told by your consultant to assess Ms Sheene first.

Task: Please speak to Ms Sheene and elicit a history with regards to her drug usage and explore more about her social circumstances. Please note that in the next station, you will need to speak to her partner to discuss the relevant management plans.

Outline of station:

You are Ms Sheene, a 31-year-old female and you are known to the drug and addiction services. You started using heroin and other drugs (such as crack) when you were a teenager. However, you have stopped using the other drugs and have been dependent on heroin mainly. You realized that you needed some help for your drug issues two years ago, and you have been on constant follow-up with the local drug and addictions service. They have previously started you on methadone. You have been on methadone for a year and have not returned to using heroin. Your current pregnancy is unplanned, and you feel a little unprepared with regards to the pregnancy. You are willing to share with the core trainee any pertinent information to help you manage your drug issues during pregnancy.

CASC Construct Table:

The CASC Construct Table is formatted so that candidates can adequately cover the range and depth of the assessment required in this station.

DOI: 10.1201/9781003313113-76

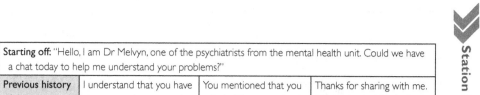

Starting off: "Hello, I am Dr Melvyn, one of the psychiatrists from the mental health unit. Could we have a chat today to help me understand your problems?"			
Previous history of drug usage and current usage	I understand that you have been seen by our service before. Could you tell me more about it?	You mentioned that you started to see us due to your usage of drugs. Can I clarify what drugs you have been using? Apart from heroin, do you use cannabis, cocaine, amphetamine, methadone, ecstasy, and sleeping tablets? Do you also use alcohol?	Thanks for sharing with me. My understanding is that you have been using heroin regularly up till last year, in that you were maintained on methadone. Could you tell me how much of methadone are you maintained on currently? Could you also share with me more about where you have been getting your methadone?
Explore methods of administration and risky behaviours	In the past, how often do you use heroin? Do you recall when was the last time you used heroin? How do you use heroin? Do you smoke it, or do you inject it?	(If the patient has been injecting) When did you first start injecting? How often do you inject? Have you shared needles previously?	How much of heroin do you use on a typical day? How much do you typically spend on your drugs?
Explore withdrawal side effects	Do you find yourself needing more heroin previously to achieve the same effects? What happens if you happen to miss your dose of heroin?	Have you experienced any side effects or withdrawal symptoms when you are not using heroin?	The typical withdrawal symptoms include that of the following: – Muscular aches – Stomach cramps – Nauseated feeling – Yawning – Rhinorrhoea
Explore the patient's feeling towards the current pregnancy	My understanding is that you have realized that you could be pregnant. How did you know?	Is this pregnancy planned or unplanned?	What are your thoughts with regard to having a child?
Exploration of Antenatal Assessment	Have you seen your antenatal doctor?	Have you undergone any scans or assessments recently?	How is the growth/size of your foetus? Did your doctor share any concerns?
Explore personal history and social circumstances	Are you currently working? Do you have any current financial difficulties?	With whom do you stay with now? How are the relationships at home?	Is there anyone who would help you care for your child at home?

Common pitfall:

a. Failure to cover the range and depth of the information required for this station.

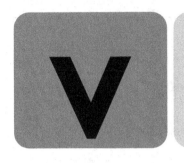

Information to candidates:

Name of patient: Ms Sheene

Ms Sheene is a 31-year-old female known previously to the drug and alcohol services as she has been using heroin since she was young. She has been maintained on methadone treatment, and she has been compliant with her methadone treatment thus far. She has missed a period for the past two months and has just discovered that she is currently pregnant. She has informed her partner about her pregnancy. Her partner, Mr Henson, is supportive and has recommended that she come by the drug and alcohol services for an evaluation as he is concerned about her continued usage of methadone during pregnancy. You are the core trainee on call and have been told by your consultant to assess Ms Sheene first. You have previously spoken to Ms Sheene, and you now have a better understanding of her drug issues. You are aware that her partner is here and wishes to see you to discuss more about the management of her addiction issues in pregnancy.

Task: Please speak to Mr Henson and address all his concerns and expectations.

Outline of station:

You are Mr Henson, the partner of Ms Sheene. You know that your partner has abused multiple drugs in the past and has been dependent on heroin for the past few years you've known her and is currently on methadone treatment. You have some questions to ask the core trainee and hope that your questions could be clarified. You want to know the risks associated with her current pregnancy since she has been on multiple drugs previously. You are concerned about how heroin and methadone might potentially harm the baby. You want to know what might happen to the baby if your partner is still abusing heroin when she is pregnant. You wonder whether it would be safe for the continuation of methadone throughout pregnancy. Also, you wish to know if your partner could breast-feed whilst she is on methadone. Lastly, in view of your partner's drug history, you are concerned that your child might be taken away from you by the social services.

CASC Construct Table:

The CASC Construct Table is formatted such that candidates would be able to cover adequately both the range and depth of the assessment required in this station.

DOI: 10.1201/9781003313113-77

Starting off: "Hello, I am Dr Melvyn, one of the psychiatrists from the mental health unit. I understand that you have some concerns about your partner and her usage of drugs. Could we have a chat about this?"			
Explanation of risk associated with drug usage in pregnancy	Could you help me to understand your concerns about your partner and her current pregnancy? Does your partner have a problem with alcohol or drug use? I think you have raised a very important issue about your partner's usage of drugs and her being pregnant at the same time. I understand your concerns about the risk associated with her drug use in pregnancy.	My understanding from speaking to your partner just now is that she used several drugs previously, and lately, she was using heroin before being maintained on methadone.	There is always the inherent risk of drugs causing issues such as stillbirth, premature delivery of the child, as well as some antenatal complications. It might also cause low birth weight. Hence, your partner must continue to see us regularly. She must also follow up and do the necessary antenatal evaluations and checks.
Safety of heroin and methadone in pregnancy	I understand that you are concerned about methadone and its effect on the current pregnancy. Please allow me to share that methadone is relatively safe in pregnancy and will not cause any abnormalities in the child.	However, should your partner continue to use heroin, it might have an impact on your child.	Previous research has shown that the usage of heroin might lead to miscarriage as well as intrauterine-related deaths.
Explanation of neonatal abstinence syndrome	One of the other effects of continued usage of heroin in pregnancy could be that of neonatal withdrawal syndrome. Have you heard of this condition before? What's your understanding of this condition? Would it be all right for me to explain more?	If your partner continues to use heroin in pregnancy, your baby might be susceptible towards acquiring neonatal withdrawal syndrome.	In essence, your baby might experience some withdrawal symptoms associated with the prior usage of heroin. We would need to monitor your baby for this. If your baby does have clinical signs and symptoms of opioid withdrawal, we might need to treat accordingly.
Explain management in pregnancy	Based on previous research findings, the best time to consider detoxification would be in the second trimester.	Methadone could still be used as a substitute and be continued throughout pregnancy.	However, there needs to be some adjustment of the dosing of methadone when your partner is in her third trimester.

(Continued)

(Continued)

Address concerns about breast-feeding and methadone	I hear your concerns with regards to the suitability of your partner breast-feeding your baby if she is on methadone.	If she is maintained on methadone at a dose of less than 20 mg/day, she could breast-feed your baby.	There are other medications that are contraindicated in breast feeding; hence, we must continue to follow up on the care of your partner and make the appropriate recommendations.
Address concerns about social services	I hear that you have some concerns about whether your child would be taken away by the social services because your partner has a drug history.	I'd like to reassure you that your child would not be taken away from you and your partner just because your partner has a drug history.	The social services would consider alternative care arrangements only under special circumstances in which it is deemed that your partner is unable to manage your child. We need your help with advising your partner to come back routinely for her appointments with us.

Common pitfall:

a. Failure to cover the range and depth of the information required for this station.

TOPIC VI

PSYCHOTHERAPIES

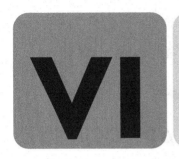

Information to candidates:

Name of patient: Mr Annis

Mr Annis is a 35-year-old male who has been referred by his GP to the mental health service as he has been having low mood with reduction of interest ever since he got dismissed from his workplace. He has been started on an antidepressant. The consultant psychiatrist has recommended that he also attend a psychotherapy session. The consultant psychiatrist wants you to share more about the specific psychotherapy (cognitive behavioural therapy) that he has recommended for the patient.

Task: Please speak to Mr Annis and counsel him with regards to how cognitive behavioural psychotherapy would work. Please also address all his expectations and concerns.

Outline of station:

You are Mr Annis, and you were diagnosed with major depressive disorder just three weeks ago and commenced on an antidepressant medication. Your mood symptoms came on following dismissal from your workplace. You understand from the consultant psychiatrist that, apart from medication, other alternatives such as psychotherapy might help you with your depressive illness. You wish to know more about the psychotherapy offered. You wish to know more about the therapy and how the therapy is structured. You also wish to know the structure of the therapy as well as the expected outcomes. You wonder whether, if therapy is effective, you could stop antidepressants as you worry about the long-term consumption of antidepressant medication.

CASC Construct Table:

The CASC Construct Table is formatted such that candidates would be able to cover adequately both the range and depth of the assessment required in this station.

DOI: 10.1201/9781003313113-78

Starting off: "Hello, I am Dr Melvyn, one of the psychiatrists from the mental health unit. I understand that you have some questions about the psychotherapy recommended. Could we have a chat about this?"			
Clarifying the nature of the therapy	I understand that the therapy that has been recommended for you is cognitive behavioural therapy (CBT). Have you heard anything about this form of psychotherapy or talking therapy before?	Cognitive behavioural therapy is a therapy that is recommended for patients with anxiety as well as depressive disorders.	It focuses on specific issues at present and does not look at past events.
Clarifying the principles of the therapy	In this form of therapy, it is believed that how we think would affect how we feel and behave. As the name suggests, it is important for you to realize that there are two main principles governing the therapy session. A total of 12 to 16 sessions are usually recommended. In the early phase, it is pertinent for the therapist to build on the therapeutic alliance. The client needs to be educated on the model of CBT and the influence of thoughts on behaviour and emotions. Goals are set for the psychotherapy session. Negative automatic thoughts are identified. The therapist would make use of questioning to reveal the self-defeating nature of the client's thought process and identify cognitive triad.	Cognitive techniques are used during the therapy session. Cognitive restructuring helps you to identify negative thoughts, dysfunctional assumptions, and maladaptive core beliefs relating to their underlying problems. It also tests the validity of those thoughts, assumptions, and beliefs. The goal is to produce more adaptive and positive alternatives. The therapist would ask the patient to keep a dysfunctional thought diary in the middle phase. The therapist would identify cognitive errors and core beliefs through the homework assignment. The therapist would practice skills for reattribution by reviewing evidence and challenging cognitive errors. Behaviour therapy involves identifying safety behaviours, entering feared situation without, safety manoeuvres, and applying relaxation	Apart from cognitive techniques, specific behavioural techniques are also used. Some of the common techniques include the following: a. Rehearsal: It helps you to anticipate challenges and to develop strategies to overcome difficulties b. Inclusion of graded assignment on exposure c. Training oneself to be self-reliant d. Pleasure and mastery of skills e. Activity scheduling to increase contact with positive activities and decrease avoidance and withdrawal f. Diversion or distraction techniques The last stage of therapy involves that of termination. The therapist would help to identify early symptoms of relapse and predict high-risk situations leading to a relapse.

(Continued)

(Continued)

		techniques, activity scheduling, and assertiveness training. The therapist would review progress and offer feedback to the client.	The client would be taught coping strategies to overcome negative emotions, interpersonal conflicts, and pressure. A plan is formulated for early intervention should a relapse take place. The skills and knowledge acquired in therapy would be consolidated.
Clarify the structure of the therapy			
Address specific concerns	Do you have any questions thus far? Is there anything else that you are concerned about with regard to the proposed therapy?	Even if there are gains in therapy and you feel better, we would not recommend that you stop your antidepressant immediately.	I know that I have shared a lot of information with you. Please allow me to offer you a brochure on cognitive behavioural therapy to help you understand more about the therapy.

Common pitfall:

a. Failure to cover the range and depth of the information required for this station.

Information to candidates:

Name of patient: Mr Patterson

You have been asked to speak to Mr Patterson. Mr Patterson is a 25-year-old footballer with the Manchester United team. Recently, in the last game, he failed to score a very important goal, resulting in the team losing the championship title. Ever since the last game, his team coach, Mark, has noticed that he is no longer able to perform on the pitch anymore and has been complaining of increased panic-like symptoms whenever he is on the pitch. Mark is very concerned about this as he used to be the star striker in the team. Mark has brought him here today for an assessment, hoping that something could be done to help him.

Task: Please speak to Mr Patterson and take a history from him. Please also try to elicit the relevant cognitive distortions that he might have.

Outline of station:

You are Mr Patterson, and your team manager, Mark, has asked you to come for a psychiatric visitation today. You failed to score an important goal in the last game in the championship last week, resulting in your team not getting the title. Ever since then, you have been feeling very anxious whenever you are on the pitch. You keep ruminating over thoughts that it was your fault, even though none of the team members have blamed you for it. In addition, even though you have been nominated as the star player for two consecutive years, you feel that it is not possible to be the star player again in view of this mistake that you have made. You feel that you are lousy on the pitch and a husband and father at home. You do not really think that the psychiatrist could do much to help you.

CASC Construct Table:

The CASC Construct Table is formatted such that candidates would be able to cover adequately both the range and depth of the assessment required in this station.

DOI: 10.1201/9781003313113-79

Starting off: "Hello, I am Dr Melvyn, one of the psychiatrists from the mental health unit. I understand that your coach requested that you see us today. Could we have a chat?"			
History of presenting complaint	Thanks for seeing us today. Could I understand from you the difficulties that you have been facing?	Thanks for sharing with me. I understand that it must have been a very difficult time for you. About the panic symptoms: Can you tell me when they first started?	Can I clarify the bodily symptoms you experience each time you have those attacks? Are there any specific thoughts that run through your mind when you are feeling so anxious? Are you worried about the next episode happening? Is there any anticipatory anxiety?
Elicit cognitive distortions of minimization and magnification	You mentioned that you have felt this way since you failed to score an important goal. I'm sorry to be hearing this. Could you tell me how you managed to play in matches prior to that miss?	It seems that you have previous successes as well. Are those previous successes not important at all? Is it true that one miss would lead to the loss of the entire match? How was the entire season like for you?	Could you have under-estimated your contribution to the team? Have you won any awards before, such as being titled the player of the year? Have you managed to score any difficult balls before? Would you not say that you were remarkable previously?
Elicit cognitive distortions of personalization and labelling	I'm sorry to learn about what happened in the last match. Who do you think is responsible for the loss?	Are you the only striker in the team? Isn't football a team sport? What about the other players? Do they not play a part in contributing to the scores? Have the other players blamed you for the recent miss in the game? It seemed to me that you attributed the team's failure solely to yourself. Could there be any other factors that might contribute to the loss of the game?	Could you tell me, what does missing a goal say about you? I hear that you're calling yourself a loser. Would you call a team-mate who merely missed one ball a loser as well?

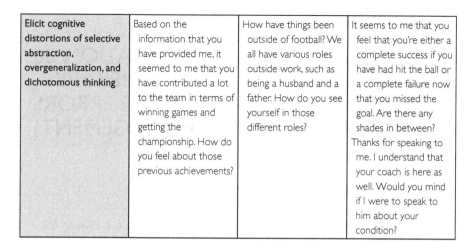

Elicit cognitive distortions of selective abstraction, overgeneralization, and dichotomous thinking	Based on the information that you have provided me, it seemed to me that you have contributed a lot to the team in terms of winning games and getting the championship. How do you feel about those previous achievements?	How have things been outside of football? We all have various roles outside work, such as being a husband and a father. How do you see yourself in those different roles?	It seems to me that you feel that you're either a complete success if you have had hit the ball or a complete failure now that you missed the goal. Are there any shades in between? Thanks for speaking to me. I understand that your coach is here as well. Would you mind if I were to speak to him about your condition?

Common pitfall:

a. Failure to cover the range and depth of the information required for this station.

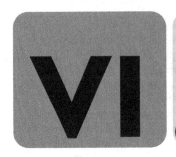

Information to candidates:

Name of patient: Mr Patterson

You have been asked to speak to Mr Patterson. Mr Patterson is a 25-year-old footballer with the Manchester United team. Recently, in the last game, he failed to score a very important goal, resulting in the team losing the championship title. Ever since the last game, his team coach, Mark, has noticed that he is no longer able to perform on the pitch and have been complaining of increased panic-like symptoms whenever he is on the pitch. Mark is very concerned about this as he used to be the star striker in the team. Mark has brought him here today for an assessment, hoping that something could be done to help him. In the previous station, you have spoken to Mr Patterson and obtained a history from him. You have managed to identify some cognitive distortions that Mr Patterson has now. You understand that Mark, his team coach, is keen to speak to you more about how he could help his player.

Task: Please speak to Mark, the team coach. Explain the presence of cognitive distortions and discuss the appropriate treatment options.

Outline of station:

You are Mark, the coach of the football team that Mr Patterson is in.

Mr Patterson has been your star player for the last two seasons. Unfortunately, he missed a very important goal during the last match, which has cost your team the championship. You do not think that it is entirely his fault as it was partly because the organization of the players on the field was suboptimal too. You realize that he has been having panic-like symptoms and have not been able to go onto the pitch. You want to know what forms of treatment could be offered to help him. You are concerned about starting him on antidepressant medication, as you are worried that the medication would impair his performance. In addition, you do not want your player to be tested positive for drugs and run afoul of the football association rules. You are concerned when the core trainee suggested starting him on a low dose of sleeping tablets to help alleviate his anxiety and panic-like symptoms.

DOI: 10.1201/9781003313113-80

CASC Construct Table:

The CASC Construct Table is formatted such that candidates would be able to cover adequately both the range and depth of the assessment required in this station.

Starting off: "Hello, I am Dr Melvyn, one of the psychiatrists from the mental health unit. I understand that you have some concerns about your player Mr Patterson. Can we have a chat about this?"			
Explanation of current assessment	I have spoken to your player previously, and I have gathered some information about his condition. He has given me his consent for me to speak to you. Could I understand from you what your concerns are with regard to your player? I fully understand your current concerns and hope I could help alleviate some of his symptoms so that he can return to the pitch as soon as possible.	Based on my assessment, it seemed like Patterson has some anxiety-like symptoms, as well as some cognitive distortions. Have you heard of the term cognitive distortions before? Let me explain more. It seems to me that he is thinking and seeing things from negative perspectives. These cognitive distortions are errors in thinking and attributions.	I sense that he is overly concerned about the goal he recently missed scoring. However, he has previous achievements, and he chooses to magnify the current problem and minimize his past achievements. Also, I realized that he has taken on all the responsibility for your team's failure to get the championship cup this season and has personalized it such that he is entirely responsible. He feels he has been a failure and has generalized these feelings to his other roles as a husband and father.
Management— pharmacological	I understand that you are very concerned how we could help him to get back to the pitch as soon as possible.	There are various options, and medication might be one option. We could start him on an antidepressant, and the one we could use would be a selective serotonin reuptake inhibitor (SSRI).	These medications would help to regulate the amount of chemical in the brain that would affect his mood and the way he thinks about things.

(Continued)

(Continued)

Management—psychological	Apart from medication, we could offer him other modalities of help.	Have you heard of this form of psychotherapy called cognitive behavioural therapy before? Cognitive behavioural therapy would be helpful for him as it focuses on his current issues, and it would help him understand how his way of thinking contributes to his feelings and behaviour.	Our therapists could help him to identify the cognitive errors he is making in his thinking. They could help him to restructure the way he thinks about things. We would usually recommend a course of therapy, and such a therapy would usually last between 12 to 16 sessions. Apart from psychological-based interventions, it is of utmost importance that your team continues to support him and provide some accommodations for him.
Address concerns	I know I have shared quite a lot of information. Do you have any questions for me?	I understand that you are quite concerned about the medication that we have recommended. Please allow me to clarify that antidepressants are not addictive in nature. Patients who are on antidepressants would not run foul of the rules of the football association as they are not performance-enhancing drugs.	We might consider giving him some hypnotics or sleeping pills to help him to alleviate his panic-like symptoms. We do need to inform you that sleeping pills are addictive in nature, and we usually do not recommend that he takes it over a protracted period.

Common pitfall:

a. Failure to cover the range and depth of the information required for this station.

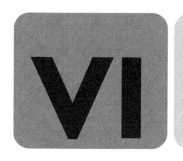

STATION 81
AGORAPHOBIA—
SYSTEMATIC
DESENSITIZATION

Information to candidates:

Name of patient: Mrs Levine

You have been tasked to speak to Mr Levine, the husband of Mrs Levine.

Mrs Levine has been seen by your consultant two weeks ago and has been diagnosed with an anxiety condition known as agoraphobia. Mr Levine is here today as he wants to know what his wife is suffering from and the causes of her current condition. He is keen to know the available treatments for her condition as well.

Task: Please speak to Mr Levine and address all his concerns and expectations.

Outline of station:

You are the husband of Mrs Levine, and you understand that your wife was seen by the psychiatrist two weeks ago. You came by today as you want to know what she is suffering from. You want to better understand what the doctors are recommending for her in terms of treatment as well. If the core trainee suggests cognitive behavioural therapy, you hope the core trainee could explain more about the therapy. In addition, you have concerns about how therapy might proceed if your wife is not amenable to step out of her house to come for the psychologist sessions.

CASC Construct Table:

The CASC Construct Table is formatted such that candidates would be able to cover adequately both the range and depth of the assessment required in this station.

DOI: 10.1201/9781003313113-81

Starting off: "Hello, I am Dr Melvyn, one of the psychiatrists from the mental health unit. I understand that you have some concerns about your wife. Could we have a chat about this?"			
Clarifying diagnosis	Could you help me to understand more about your concerns about your wife? Has any doctor told you what she is suffering from?	We have seen your wife previously and assessed her condition. It seems to us that she is suffering from a condition known as agoraphobia. Have you heard of this condition before?	Basically, agoraphobia is an anxiety condition in which the patient has anxiety-like panic symptoms, usually when they are in situations in which they perceive to be dangerous or uncomfortable. During those episodes, their fight and flight response are heightened, and they might experience an increase in heart rate/blood pressure. This is a common anxiety-related disorder and could be treated.
Explaining pharmacological treatment	There are several options with regards to treatment. We could start by helping your wife understand more about anxiety and more about her condition.	We do recommend a course of antidepressants to help her with her condition.	Antidepressant would help in the regulation of brain chemicals that are involved in anxiety state and would be beneficial for your wife. At times, we might consider the short-term prescription of anti-anxiety medication (for individuals with severe anxiety symptoms).
Explaining psychological treatment	Apart from medication, your wife might benefit from a form of talking therapy called cognitive behavioural therapy. Have you heard about this form of therapy before?	In this form of therapy, it is believed that how we think would affect how we feel and behave. As the name suggests, it is important for you to realize that there are two main principles governing the therapy session.	Cognitive techniques are used during the therapy session. Apart from cognitive techniques, specific behavioural techniques are also used. Some of the common behavioural techniques that might be helpful for your wife include that of breathing exercises as well as relaxation training. One component of this therapy that is highly effective is that of systematic desensitization (SD).

Clarifying the structure of treatment	In SD, this usually refers to graded exposure with relaxation. It involves allowing your wife to draw up a hierarchy of her fears and then involving her performing the less anxiety-provoking behaviours first and then progressing on to those that are more anxiety-provoking. The therapist would pair this together with relaxation exercises.	The total duration of therapy might take up to 12 to 16 sessions. We will arrange for your wife to meet up with the therapist on a weekly basis. Each session usually last for around 45 minutes to an hour. There might be some homework exercises prescribed in between the sessions.	The therapist might go through the homework exercises in the initial part of the session. They might also go through some of the core skills reviewed in the previous session.
Address concerns and expectations	I know that I have shared quite a lot of information. Do you have any questions for me now?	I hear your concerns about how therapy could potentially progress if your wife cannot afford to come out of the house. We might be able to make some arrangements for the therapist to visit your wife at home to get the therapy started.	I understand that you have heard that Valium might be useful for her condition. It is a hypnotic medication and could be useful for her to calm her down, but over the longer term, we are concerned about its addictive potential. With regards to antidepressants, they are not addictive in nature. I would like to offer you a brochure about CBT and SD. Please feel free to contact myself if you need further clarification.

Common pitfalls:

a. Failure to cover the range and depth of the information required for this station.

b. Failure to explain anxiety disorder in layman's terms.

c. Failure to explain core aspects of the therapy in layman's terms.

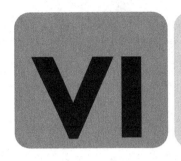

STATION 82
OCD—EXPOSURE AND RESPONSE PREVENTION

Information to candidates:

Name of patient: Mr Alders

You have been tasked to speak to Mr Alders, who has been referred by his GP for excessive hand washing. Your consultant has diagnosed him with obsessive-compulsive disorder. He has defaulted a follow-up appointment with your consultant but is here today seeking help. He has not taken the antidepressant prescribed previously and is worried about being on medication. He hopes that you can offer an alternative to medication. He has read up online and heard that there are some psychological treatments for his condition. He wants to know more about them.

Task: Please speak to Mr Alders and discuss with him more about psychological treatment, in particular, the specific form of behaviour therapy that might be indicated in his case. Please address all his concerns and expectations.

Outline of station:

You are Mr Alders, and you have been referred previously by your GP to see the psychiatrist because of your excessive preoccupation with contamination and needing to wash because of your preoccupations. The psychiatrist has diagnosed you with obsessive-compulsive disorder and has recommended a course of antidepressants. You are ambivalent about being on medication and have not started on the medication recommended by the consultant psychiatrist. You have searched for more information about your condition on the Internet, and you realize that there are alternatives to medication, such as psychological treatment. You wish to know more about the appropriate psychological treatment. You hope that the doctor you're seeing today can give you a better overview of psychological treatment.

CASC Construct Table:

The CASC Construct Table is formatted such that candidates would be able to cover adequately both the range and depth of the assessment required in this station.

DOI: 10.1201/9781003313113-82

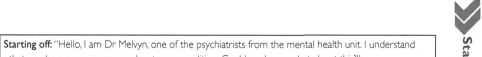

Starting off: "Hello, I am Dr Melvyn, one of the psychiatrists from the mental health unit. I understand that you have some concerns about your condition. Could we have a chat about this?"			
Discuss alternatives to medication	I understand that my consultant has seen you recently and has started you on an antidepressant medication. Could I understand your concerns about your current condition?	I hear your concerns about being on medication (antidepressants) for your condition. Please let me share with you that antidepressant is not addictive in nature. We do usually prescribe an antidepressant for patients who are suffering from similar condition as yours.	I hear that you wish to consider alternatives to medication. There are alternatives such as psychotherapy for your current condition. Have you heard of this therapy known as cognitive behavioural therapy before? Could you share with me more about your understanding of this form of therapy?
Explanation about cognitive aspects of CBT	In this form of therapy, it is believed that how we think affects how we feel and behave. As the name suggests, it is important for you to realize that there are two main principles governing the therapy session. Apart from the cognitive component of this form of therapy, other behavioural techniques are used in this form of therapy. You might be taught relaxation techniques such as deep breathing or progressive muscle relaxation. These techniques help not only in managing the fears that drive your anxiety but also help you to better manage the physical symptoms associated with your anxiety.	Cognitive techniques are used during the therapy session. One form of behavioural therapy, known as exposure and response prevention, is very helpful for your condition. Do you have any ideas about what it entails?	Cognitive restructuring helps you to identify negative thoughts, dysfunctional assumptions, and maladaptive core beliefs relating to their underlying problems. It also tests the validity of those thoughts, assumptions, and beliefs. The goal is to produce more adaptive and positive alternatives. Exposure and response prevention involves first making a hierarchy of situations from the least anxious to the most anxious provoking. The therapist will gradually expose you to the situation to which you are fearful of being in and, at the same time, will prevent you from performing your routine ritual.

(Continued)

(Continued)

Explanation about behavioural aspects of CBT			This allows the individual to discover what happens when they do not perform the rituals typically associated with compulsions.
Explain structure of sessions	The total duration of therapy might range between 12 to 16 sessions.	Each session would usually last between 45 minutes to an hour. There might be some homework that is being assigned in between the sessions.	You will be engaging with a therapist who has professional training in this area.
Address other concerns and expectations	I know that I have shared a whole of information. Do you have any questions for me?	CBT, and in particular, exposure and response prevention therapy, has been known to be efficacious for patients with obsessive-compulsive disorder.	I'd like to offer you some brochures to take home, for you to understand more about what psychological therapy entails. Would that be all right with you? Should you have any other questions, please feel free to fix a time with me for further discussion.

Common pitfall:

a. Failure to cover the range and depth of the information required for this station.

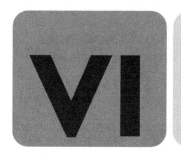

STATION 83 PANIC DISORDER AND HYPERVENTILATION (PATIENT MANAGEMENT)

Information to candidates:

Name of patient: Mr Winslow

You have been asked to review a 40-year-old male, Mr Winslow, in the emergency room. Your medical colleagues have informed you that Mr Winslow came through the emergency services as he called the ambulance after feeling unwell at home. He told the medics that he felt as if he was having a heart attack. The medics have done the necessary biochemical investigation and heart tracing monitoring and have ruled out an underlying cardiac issue. The medics strongly believe that Mr Winslow is feeling this way due to possibly an underlying psychiatric disorder. Apart from the normal results obtained thus far, the medics are convinced that he does not have a cardiac history as the cardiologist in the outpatient clinic has extensively worked him up. You have been informed that Mr Winslow has a positive family history of cardiovascular disease; in fact, two of his relatives just passed on recently due to cardiac arrest. His daughter, Sarah, is here and wants to speak to you. She is deeply concerned about her father's issue.

Task: Please speak to Sarah, the daughter of Mr Winslow, and explain the likely diagnosis for him. Please also address all her concerns and expectations accordingly.

Outline of station:

You are the daughter of Mr Winslow, and you are quite distressed by your father's condition. This is the fifth time he has called an ambulance to take him to the hospital this month. You are especially worried as two of your close relatives have just passed on due to underlying cardiac issues. You understand that the cardiologist has extensively worked up your father, and thus far there have not been any abnormalities discovered. You are curious about what is wrong with your father now that he has been referred to a psychiatrist. If the core trainee explains that he might have an underlying panic disorder or hyperventilation disorder, you expect the core trainee to explain more about the disorders. You want to know from the core trainee how best you as a carer could help support his current condition. You wonder whether there is any role for medication in his case. In addition, you wonder whether your father would be fit for his regular routine of golfing.

DOI: 10.1201/9781003313113-83

CASC Construct Table:

The CASC Construct Table is formatted such that candidates would be able to cover adequately both the range and depth of the assessment required in this station.

Starting off: "Hello, I am Dr Melvyn, one of the psychiatrists from the mental health unit. I understand that you have some concerns about your father's condition. Could we have a chat about it?"			
Explanation of current findings and reassurance	I'm sorry to hear how difficult it has been for you. I understand that you are very worried about your father's condition. My emergency room colleagues have informed me to see your father and how we could jointly help your father.	Based on my understanding, the medical team have done quite a comprehensive evaluation of his medical condition. So far, the laboratory investigations that have been done are normal, and the heart tracing is also normal.	The medical team does not think that your father has un underlying heart condition or that he is having a heart attack. From my understanding, he has been seen by the cardiologist recently, who has also done a very comprehensive workup. Thus far, everything seemed fine with regards to his heart.
Clarify diagnosis of panic disorder	I hear that you're concerned about the underlying cause, given that all the investigations done are normal. This is the reason why my medical colleagues have called upon me. At times, some patients with psychiatric condition might experience such symptoms. Would you mind if I go on to explain more after having spoken to and having assessed your father?	One of the conditions that we feel your father might have now is that of a panic disorder. Have you heard of panic disorders before? Could I go on to explain more about panic disorder? Panic disorder usually involves recurrent unpredictable attacks of severe anxiety lasting for only a few minutes.	There could be a sudden onset of palpitations, chest pain, choking, dizziness, depersonalization, and derealization, together with a fear of dying, losing control, or going mad. It often results in a hurried exit and a subsequent avoidance of similar situations. This is in turn followed by persistent fears of another attack.

Clarify the diagnosis of hyperventilation disorder	The other clinical diagnosis that we think your father could have is hyperventilation syndrome. Have you heard about this condition before?	Hyperventilation syndrome results when an individual makes excessive use of accessory muscles to breathe, thus resulting in hyper-inflated lungs.	The symptoms of hyperventilation disorder can resemble that of panic disorder.
Management	There are various ways we could help to manage your father's symptoms.	The acute phase usually involves reassuring patients and helping them establish normal breathing patterns. Sometimes, the anxiety can be reduced through the prescription of anxiolytics.	In the longer term, the management involves teaching appropriate relaxation techniques. If the condition persists, we could consider referring your father for a form of psychotherapy or talking therapy known as cognitive behavioural therapy (CBT). Have you heard of this therapy before? Could I leave you a brochure about the therapy for you to understand the therapy further?
Address all concerns and expectations	I understand that I have shared quite a lot of information. Do you have any specific questions you wish to clarify or ask?	With regards to medication, there are some medications available to help with his anxiety condition, apart from the hypnotics we have discussed earlier. At times, we do consider the commencement of antidepressants to help with the symptoms.	With time, I am hopeful that your father would respond well to the treatment, and he should be able to get back to activities he used to enjoy previously.

Common pitfall:

a. Failure to cover the range and depth of the information required for this station.

Information to candidates:

Name of patient: Ms Grant

You have been tasked to see Ms Grant, a 25-year-old female who has been referred to the specialist service by her GP. The GP noted that she has been low in her mood following the loss of her mother, as well as due to her relationship issues with her husband. The consultant psychiatrist has previously recommended a combination of medication as well as interpersonal psychotherapy, but she was not keen. However, she is back here for a follow-up, and she is keen to consider interpersonal psychotherapy. She hopes to find out more about the therapy prior to commencing on it.

Task: Please speak to Ms Grant and explain more about interpersonal psychotherapy to her. Please assess to see if she is suitable for the therapy. If she is not suitable for the therapy, please recommend other alternatives for her.

Outline of station:

You are Ms Grant, a 25-year-old female who has been referred to the specialist service by your GP. The consultant psychiatrist has previously recommended a combination of medication and interpersonal psychotherapy for your depressive symptoms. However, you were not keen on psychotherapy. You have returned today as you feel that you are more ready for it. Your recent stressors include the recent loss of your beloved mother, as well as some relationship issues with your husband. Recently, there have been some changes at the workplace as well as your company is streamlining the business and are dismissing some staff. You would like to know more about the therapy and whether it would be suitable for you.

CASC Construct Table:

The CASC Construct Table is formatted such that candidates would be able to cover adequately both the range and depth of the assessment required in this station.

DOI: 10.1201/9781003313113-84

Starting off: "Hello, I am Dr Melvyn, one of the psychiatrists from the mental health unit. I understand that you have some concerns. Could we have a chat about it?"			
History of presenting complaint	I understand that you have been seen by our consultant and have been diagnosed with depression. How long have you been feeling low for? When did this first start?	Apart from your low mood, do you find yourself having less interest in things or activities which you previously enjoy doing? How is your energy level like? Do you have enough energy to get through a normal day?	How has your sleep been for you? What about your appetite? Could you manage your meals? Have things been so stressful for you that you have had unusual experiences (such as hearing voices) when you are alone? Have you felt that life is no longer worth living? Have you entertained thoughts recently with regard to ending your life?
Determination of whether her current symptoms are suitable for interpersonal psychotherapy	Did the consultant psychiatrist explain to you what mental health condition you have? Did he inform you more about the severity of your mental health condition?	Prior to this, have you seen a psychiatrist?	Interpersonal therapy is usually indicated for patients with mild to moderate depression and not for patients with bipolar disorder or severe depression. Therefore I am checking with you your past history.
Identify recent grief	Could you share with me your recent stressors? I am sorry to learn that your mother has passed on recently.	How have you been coping with the loss? Was it a sudden event, or did you have knowledge that your mother has been ill for some time?	Did you manage to attend the funeral? How are you feeling with regard to your mother's death currently?
Identify interpersonal disputes	Besides the recent loss of your mother, have there been any other matters that have been bothering you?	Could you tell me a bit more about how your relationship with your husband has been bothering you?	How long has it been bothering you? Apart from the frequent disagreements and arguments, has your husband been physically aggressive towards you?

(Continued)

(Continued)

Identify role transitions	Have there been any other changes in your life?	You mentioned that there have been some changes at your workplace. Could you tell me more?	
Identify interpersonal role deficits	Is there someone to whom you could confide in when you feel low in your mood?	How is your relationship with your family members?	What about your relationships with your friends and colleagues?
Explanation of structure of therapy	The main aim of IPT is to reduce your suffering and to improve interpersonal functioning. IPT focuses mainly on the interpersonal relationship as a means to bring about change. The goal is to help you to improve your interpersonal relationships or change your expectations on interpersonal relationship.	IPT is designed to help you to recognize your interpersonal needs and to seek attachment and reassurance in the process of improving interpersonal relationship.	There are three main stages of IPT. In the first stage, the therapist would try their best to develop a good therapeutic relationship with you and to understand your problems. In the second stage, the therapist will analyse the way you communicate with other people. The therapist will give you useful advice and help you develop new skills through role-play. In the final stage, the therapist will strengthen the skills you learned in the therapy. The therapist will help to identify resources for you to handle interpersonal problems in the future. The whole IPT takes around 16–20 sessions.

Common pitfalls:

a. Failure to cover the range and depth of the information required for this station.

b. Failure to demonstrate concepts related to IPT, such as loss in role and grief, role transitions, role disputes, and role-play.

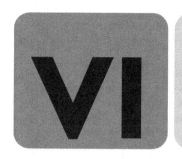

Information to candidates:

Name of patient: Mr Allsop
   You have been asked to see Mr Allsop, who has requested to stop attending his psychotherapy sessions. He has been enrolled in psychodynamic psychotherapy and has attended three sessions.

Task: Please speak to him and explore his reasons for wanting to discontinue therapy. Please advise him accordingly.

Outline of station:
   You are Mr Allsop, and you were diagnosed with depression around two months ago. The psychiatrist recommends for you to be on an antidepressant as well as to commence psychotherapy. You have attended three sessions of psychotherapy, but you are reluctant to continue with therapy. You do not think you wish to continue, although you know your depressive symptoms have not actually improved. There have not been any other changes in life causing you to want to terminate therapy. You do not have any financial concerns that would limit your attendance at psychotherapy. You wish to stop the current therapy as you do not wish to be constantly talking about your past. You feel that the therapist is cold and unemotional and not understanding, and he seems to be critical towards you sometimes. This brings to mind some past relationships you have had. You are not keen to continue with therapy no matter what the core trainee says.

CASC Construct Table:

The CASC Construct Table is formatted such that candidates would be able to cover adequately both the range and depth of the assessment required in this station.

DOI: 10.1201/9781003313113-85

Starting off: "Hello, I am Dr Melvyn, one of the psychiatrists from the mental health unit. I understand that you have some concerns with regards to the therapy that you are attending. Could we have a chat about it?"

Exploration of potential reasons leading to discontinuation of therapy—patient factors	I understand that you have some concerns about the therapy that has been recommended and organized for you. Can you help me understand more about it? How many sessions of therapy have you attended thus far?	At times, patients tell us that they wish to discontinue therapy for various reasons. Sometimes, it is because they feel that therapy has been going on well for them and their symptoms have improved. Is this the case for you? How have you been feeling in your mood?	Patients sometimes wish to discontinue therapy as they have experienced some changes in their life. Have there been any recent changes in your life? Have you moved house recently? Is there adequate time for you to attend the therapy sessions? Do you have financial concerns that might limit your attendance?
Exploration of potential reasons leading to discontinuation of therapy—therapist factors	Thanks for sharing your concerns with me. Sometimes, patients tell us they wish to discontinue therapy for therapist-related reasons.	Have you ever felt that your therapist is not competent enough to help you with your problems? Do you feel that they lacks the necessary competence and experience?	Is one of the reasons for you wanting to discontinue therapy that you do not have trust in the therapist? You mentioned that you have undergone three psychotherapy sessions thus far. Has there been any therapist change in between the sessions you have attended thus far?
Identification of core problems	You mentioned that you do not feel comfortable with the therapist. Would you mind telling me more? In what ways does the therapist make you feel uncomfortable?	I'm sorry to hear that you feel that the therapist seemed to be critical towards you. You also mentioned that the therapist seemed cold and unemotional throughout the therapy sessions.	Does the attitude of the therapist remind you of any previous relationships you have had? Can you tell me more? Am I right to say that the way you are currently feeling toward the therapist is like the way you used to feel towards your father (to whom you felt was very harsh and critical towards you)?

Explanation of transference	It seems to me that the way you feel towards the therapist is due to transference. Have you heard about this before?	Transference is the process in which a patient projects onto the therapist feelings and emotions that are derived from previous difficult relationships (in your case, it seemed to me that the previous difficult relationship you have had was that with your father).	Whilst transference might seem to limit the therapy, it is also crucial to work through these feelings.
Address concerns and advise patient accordingly	I understand that you are not keen to continue with therapy. However, I hope that you could reconsider this. Sometimes we advise our patients that when they are undergoing psychotherapy, they might feel worse before getting better.	It is important for you to speak to your therapist more about the feelings that you are having now, as it is important to address and work through these feelings as it might affect your future relationships with others.	Do you have any questions for me? I really hope you can reconsider and speak to your therapist. Of course, should you still feel strongly against therapy, we could arrange another session to discuss further how best we could help you with regards to the therapy.

Common pitfalls:

a. Failure to cover the range and depth of the information required for this station.

b. Failure to explore all possible areas for patient's wish to terminate therapy.

**Do not appear to be paternalistic in the approach of this station. Explore the patient's concerns and expectations and respect their decision.

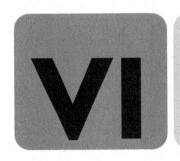

Information to candidates:

Name of patient: Mr Moss

You have been tasked to Mr Moss, who is a 40-year-old male whom his GP has referred. His GP has stated in the memo that Mr Moss has been having many difficulties at work. He is having difficulties meeting the datelines at work and in terms of his relationship with his work colleagues.

Task: Please speak to Mr Moss with the aim of understanding more about his difficulties at work. Please identify the relevant psychodynamic defences that he may be using. You are expected to explain to the patient more about his condition and address all his concerns and expectations.

Outline of station:

You are Mr Moss, a 40-year-old male whom your GP has referred for having difficulties at work. Recently, you have been having difficulties with work, especially in terms of your relationships with your colleagues. You have been married for two months, and things have not gone well with your current marital relationship. Your wife is keen to have a child, but you are not feeling prepared about it. You have been trying to explain to her, but it always ends up in an argument. You are not sure why this is affecting your work as well. Your colleagues have mentioned that you appeared more irritable when you are working with them. You have decided to see your GP as you realized that you needed some help.

CASC Construct Table:

The CASC Construct Table is formatted such that candidates would be able to cover adequately both the range and depth of the assessment required in this station.

DOI: 10.1201/9781003313113-86

Starting off: "Hello, I am Dr Melvyn, one of the psychiatrists from the mental health unit. I understand that you have been referred by your GP for work-related difficulties. Could we have a chat about this?"			
History of presenting history	I understand from the memo that you have seen your GP for work-related difficulties. Could you tell me more about what has been troubling you at work?	I'm sorry to be hearing about this. It must have been a difficult time for you. Did your colleagues comment about the change in your work attitude as well?	How long has this been for you, that you have been having difficulties at work?
Current stressor	How has your mood been recently? Have you lost interest in things which you have previously enjoyed doing? Is there anything that is bothering you now?	Have there been any problems at home with regards to finances or relationships? Can you tell me more?	I'm sorry to hear that things have been difficult for you at home. You mentioned that there had been some difficulties in terms of your relationship with your wife. Does that result in frequent arguments? How has she been treating you currently?
Identification of relevant psychodynamic defences that patient is using	You seem to have been undergoing a very tough period for the last two months. Things have not been going well since you got married. You have been quite upset about your wife.	There is a chance that your current difficulties with your work and in terms of your relationship with your colleague might result from your difficulties at home.	Sometimes, when we are undergoing stressful situations, we tend to displace and shift our emotions from one situation onto another situation. For example, a colleague whom the consultant might have scolded for her performance might project her anger towards her family members or an object. This is common and is a form of a defence mechanism known as displacement. Have you heard of this before?
Address concerns and expectations	I understand that your work-related issues are additional stress for you.	I hope I can refer you to the counsellor or perhaps the psychotherapist for them to help you cope with the situation better.	Would that be fine for you? Do you have any other questions for me?

Common pitfall:

   a. Failure to cover the range and depth of the information required for this station.

**In this station, you may want to consider using the technique of "reflection," using examples that the patient cited to reflect the core defence mechanism. This will help demonstrate to the examiner that you are doing a systematic interview and know the defence mechanisms.

TOPIC VII

EATING DISORDERS

Information to candidates:

Name of patient: Ms Yan

You have been tasked to see Ms Yan, a 20-year-old female whom her GP has referred. During the recent routine health screening with her GP, her GP noted that her BMI is on the lower limit. Ms Yan did share that she has been restricting her diet to achieve the desired body weight. The GP has referred her to your service as the GP felt that Ms Yan would benefit from some form of help for her eating issues. She has been admitted to the inpatient unit, and her weight has stabilized after commencing gradual re-feeding. The psychologist is due to see her today but would like to know more about her background and the prognostic factors for her.

Task: Please speak to Ms Yan and elicit both the positive and negative prognostic factors.

Outline of station:

You are Ms Yan, and your GP initially referred you to the mental health service. You have been admitted to the inpatient unit since. The team has commenced gradually re-feeding, and your weight has improved. You are due to see a psychologist. You understand that the core trainee is supposed to speak to you to get more information about the prognostic factors regarding your condition. You will share the following information with the core trainee: You have had this disorder since the age of 14, but you have had only one hospitalization since then. There were times when you have had bingeing behaviours, such as vomiting and purging. Your relationship with your family is not good. You do not have any other comorbid psychiatric history.

CASC Construct Table:

The CASC Construct Table is formatted such that candidates would be able to cover adequately both the range and depth of the assessment required in this station.

DOI: 10.1201/9781003313113-87

Starting off: "Hello, I am Dr Melvyn, one of the psychiatrists from the mental health unit. I understand that you have been admitted to the inpatient unit recently. Could we have a chat?"			
Explore the longitudinal history of symptoms	I understand that you have been diagnosed with anorexia nervosa. Could you tell me more about it?	Do you remember at what age you were diagnosed with this disorder?	Were you diagnosed before the age of 15 years old? Have you had any previous hospital stay for your symptoms?
Explore core symptoms for AN	Do you remember what your weight was when you were first diagnosed?	Could you tell me more about your anorexia symptoms?	Did you suffer from any physical complications because of anorexia nervosa symptoms? Did you have any difficulties with your menstrual cycle? How long did these difficulties last for you? How long was it before you went ahead to seek help?
Explore the presence of bulimic features	Apart from the symptoms that you have mentioned, have you had any of these symptoms since the time you were diagnosed?	Do you have a persistent preoccupation with eating and an irresistible craving for food, with episodes of overeating in which large amounts of food are consumed in short periods of time?	Have you ever made any attempts to counteract the fattening effects of food using one or more of the following: self-induced vomiting, purgative abuse, alternating periods of starvation, or the usage of drugs?
Explore social circumstances	How is your current relationship with your family?	Is your family supportive? Or are there continued family problems?	Do your parents set unrealistic expectations for you?
Explore psychiatric comorbidities	Have you had any other consultations with a psychiatrist for other mental health problems?	Do you have any family history of mental health problems?	How would you describe yourself in terms of your personality? Are you perfectionistic? Do you feel that you could be impulsive at times?

Common pitfall:

a. Failure to cover the range and depth of the information required for this station.

Information to candidates:

Name of patient: Ms Alcazar

You have been asked to speak to Ms Alcazar, a 25-year-old female. She has been referred by her GP to the mental health service. She has visited her GP as she has been missing her menstrual periods for the last two months. The GP managed to gather more information from her and realized that she had been intentionally losing weight for the past year or so.

Task: Please speak to Ms Alcazar and get a history to establish a diagnosis. Please also assess for aetiological factors.

Outline of station:

You are Ms Alcazar, a 25-year-old university student, and your GP has referred you to the mental health service. You have been told by your GP that you are likely to be having a weight problem. It is true that over the past couple of months, you have been trying to lose as much weight as possible to get to your ideal weight. You have been exercising excessively and have been skipping meals at times as well. You have another sister who has an eating disorder as well. Since you were young, you have been a perfectionistic person. You do not have any other comorbid psychiatric disorders.

CASC Construct Table:

The CASC Construct Table is formatted such that candidates would be able to cover adequately both the range and depth of the assessment required in this station.

DOI: 10.1201/9781003313113-88

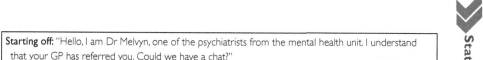

Starting off: "Hello, I am Dr Melvyn, one of the psychiatrists from the mental health unit. I understand that your GP has referred you. Could we have a chat?"			
Explore core symptoms	I understand that your GP has referred you to see us. Could you tell me more? I'm sorry to learn of the circumstances of the referral. I like to understand more about your symptoms to help you with your weight issues. Can you tell me your average weight over the past couple of months? What was your highest and lowest weight over the past couple of months? Do you have an ideal weight that you are targeting? What is your ideal weight?	Could you share with me what methods you have been adopting to lose weight? Do you tend to avoid food? Do you engage in excessive exercise? Have you tried to induce vomiting before? Do you use laxatives or diuretics to help you lose weight? Have you tried any other methods to lose weight?	Do you constantly think about food? Do you find yourself counting the calories of the food that you eat? How do you feel about your body? Do you constantly think that you are too fat? Has anyone questioned you about the way you have been feeling?
Explore complications arising from AN diagnosis	I'm sorry but I need to ask you some personal questions. Could you tell me more about your periods? Have they been regular? Are they affected at all?	Have you ever had any other complications in view of your low weight? Have you ever felt faint or dizzy before? Do you feel weak most of the time?	Have you required any hospitalization due to these medical issues?
Explore aetiological factors	Could you tell me more about your family? Are your family members close to you? Do you think that you have been too close to them?	How is the relationship between yourself and your siblings? Do you have anyone in the family with an eating disorder?	How do illnesses affect the dynamics in the family? Do you tend to get more attention from the rest of the family? How do you think your family will react when they learn that you have an eating disorder? What is your family's view on food and body image? Finally, can you tell me more about your childhood? What was it like? Is there anything that sticks out? Could you also briefly tell me more about your personality?

(Continued)

Rule out other psychiatric comorbidities	How has your mood been lately? Are you still interested in doing things you were previously interested in doing?	How have your energy levels been? How has your sleep been? Can you focus and concentrate on things you like to do?	Have you had any unusual experiences, such as hearing voices when no one is there? Do you feel that life is meaningless and not worth living?

Common pitfall:

a. Failure to cover the range and depth of the information required for this station.

Information to candidates:

Name of patient: Ms Alcazar

You have been asked to speak to Ms Alcazar, a 25-year-old female. Her GP has referred her to the mental health service. She has visited her GP as she has been missing her menstrual periods for the past two months. The GP managed to gather more information from her and realized that she had been intentionally losing weight for the past year or so. You have previously spoken to her to come to a diagnosis. You have also obtained further history regarding relevant aetiological factors. In addition, you have a medical student who is attached to the team, and the student is keen to understand more about the diagnosis, factors predisposing her to the disorder, and the management approach.

Task: Please explain the diagnosis and clarify the aetiological factors predisposing her to her current condition. Please also discuss the most appropriate treatment plans.

Outline of station:

You are the medical student who is attached to the team and have heard about this case from the psychiatry consultant on call. You understand that one of the trainees has assessed her, and you like to know more about the assessment.

CASC Construct Table:

The CASC Construct Table is formatted such that candidates would be able to cover adequately both the range and depth of the assessment required in this station.

DOI: 10.1201/9781003313113-89

Starting off: "Hello, I am Dr Melvyn, one of the core trainees from the mental health unit. I understand that you have some questions about the patient that I just saw. Could we have a chat?"			
Clarification of diagnosis	I have just seen Ms Alcazar, a 25-year-old female whom her GP has referred. She has been restricting her diet for the past couple of months to achieve ideal body weight. Based on the history I have obtained, the main diagnosis I suspect now is that of anorexia nervosa. Have you heard of the term anorexia nervosa before? (Or) What is your understanding of this condition?	Please allow me to share more about the condition. Anorexia nervosa is characterized by deliberate weight loss, thus resulting in undernutrition and resultant endocrine and metabolic disturbances. The following needs to be present for us to make the diagnosis: a. Significantly low body weight (less than what is minimally normal) b. There must be weight loss self-induced by the avoidance of fattening food by methods such as self-induced vomiting, excessive exercise, and use of appetite suppressants. c. Body image distortion.	Usually, the peak age of onset of these symptoms are around 15 to 19 years old. The incidence of this condition is ten times higher in females as compared to males. The condition is usually more prevalent in the higher socio-economic classes.
Explain common aetiological factors	There are multiple factors that might predispose an individual towards this condition. If there is a family history of this condition, she will be at an increased risk of acquiring the disorder.	Several studies have also demonstrated the involvement of brain chemicals (dopamine) in this condition. An excess of physical illness in childhood may also predispose individuals towards the development of the condition. For some individuals, childhood obesity might also be a predisposing factor.	Psychological factors might also predispose an individual towards the disorder. In addition, those who have obsessive and impulsive traits are at enhanced risk for developing the disorder as well. In addition, family relationships might also predispose an individual towards an eating disorder. A typical anorexic usually comes from an inward, often overprotected and highly controlled family. The culture of thinness might also be a predisposing factor.

Explain treatment options	Before starting any treatment, baseline vitals and laboratory work need to be done.	Most individuals with this condition could be treated on an outpatient basis. Inpatient care is indicated for patients who are very emaciated. There are a variety of treatment options available, to which I will elaborate on further. We need to get the dietician involved and aim for an average weekly gain of 0.5 kg to 1 kg. The dietician could also provide advice about re-feeding, in order to avoid re-feeding syndromes.	Apart from medication, psychotherapy could be of benefit. Cognitive behavioural therapy, cognitive analytic therapy, interpersonal therapy, and focal and even family interventions that focuses explicitly on eating disorders. CBT largely targets the cognitive distortions and behaviours related to body weight, body image, and eating. Based on the NICE recommendations, outpatient psychological treatment should be offered after discharge, and the duration is for at least 12 months. Usually, medication is not used as the sole or primary treatment for AN.
Clarify any concerns	I understand that you have some concerns about the prognosis of the patient. Could I share more about her prognosis?	Her prognosis would be considered good if she has the following prognostic factors: Onset prior to the age of 15; higher weight at onset and at presentation; having received treatment within three months after the onset of illness; recovery within two years after initiation of treatment; supportive family; has the motivation to change along with good children social adjustment.	Her prognosis will be considered poor if she has the following prognostic factors: Onset at older age; lower weight at onset and at presentation; very frequent vomiting and presence of bulimia; very severe weight loss, long duration of AN; previous hospitalization; extreme resistance to treatment; continued family problems.

Common pitfall:

a. Failure to cover the range and depth of the information required for this station.

Information to candidates:

Name of patient: Ms Ravenhill

You have been tasked to see Ms Rebecca Ravenhill, a 20-year-old university student. She has a history of type I diabetes mellitus and has been recommended to be on long-term subcutaneous insulin injection. Recently, she has been admitted to the hospital twice following episodes of hyperglycaemia. The medics have been concerned about her recurrent admissions. She did share with the medics that she has frequently been omitting insulin as she has an ideal body weight and size and is trying to achieve that. The medics have decided to get your opinion about her case.

Task: Please speak to Ms Ravenhill and elicit an eating disorder history with the aim of concluding what subtype of eating disorder she is suffering from. Please also assess for both positive and negative prognostic factors as it will have an impact on further treatment.

Outline of station:

You are Ms Rebecca Ravenhill, a 20-year-old university student. You have an intense morbid fear of fatness. You have persistent food craving approximately three times a week and would indulge in binge eating. After your binge eating, you would resort to measures to lose weight, such as avoidance of foods and fluids as well as vomiting. You have a history of depression, and you have had these symptoms for the last five years. Your premorbid personality is that you are very introverted with low self-esteem.

CASC Construct Table:

The CASC Construct Table is formatted such that candidates would be able to cover adequately both the range and depth of the assessment required in this station.

DOI: 10.1201/9781003313113-90

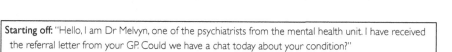

Starting off: "Hello, I am Dr Melvyn, one of the psychiatrists from the mental health unit. I have received the referral letter from your GP. Could we have a chat today about your condition?"			
Eating disorder history	Could you please tell me more about what has been troubling you? I understand from your GP that you have been having some issues with your diet? Could you tell me more? Can you share with me your height, weight, and your current body mass index (BMI)?	Do you find yourself being overly preoccupied with eating and having irresistible craving for food? Have there been episodes to which you overeat large amount of food in a short period of time? How frequently does this occur for you?	After your binge episodes, do you indulge in any attempt to try to counteract the fattening effects of food? Have you resorted to self-induced vomiting and misuse of purgative? I understand that you have an underlying diabetic condition. Have there been times you have missed out on your insulin dose? Could you tell me why you decided to miss your regular doses? Is there an ideal weight that you are trying to achieve? Do you have an ideal BMI that you are trying to achieve?
Eliciting psychological symptoms	What are your thoughts with regard to your body image? Are you very concerned that you are fat?	Could you tell me more about your emotions before and after your binge-eating episodes?	Do you try to restrict the amount of food you take? Do you engage in excessive exercise?
Eliciting physical signs and complications	Sometimes, patients do have bodily symptoms because of their eating problems.	Have you had any bodily symptoms?	

(Continued)

(Continued)

Assessing prognostic factors	Have you seen a psychiatrist before? What did the psychiatrist diagnose you with? Do you have anyone in your family who has a mental health–related disorder?	Do you remember when your symptoms first started? Have you required any hospitalizations as a result of your eating habits?	Could you tell me more about your personality? Were there any problems previously when you were younger? How was your childhood like? Have you had issues with your interpersonal relationships? Are most of your relationships relatively intense and short? Do you feel a sense of abandonment in between these relationships? Have you self-harmed or attempted suicide before? Do you use any other substances like alcohol or drugs to cope with stressors in life?

Common pitfall:

a. Failure to cover the range and depth of the information required for this station.

STATION 91
RE-FEEDING SYNDROME AND USE OF MENTAL HEALTH ACT (PATIENT MANAGEMENT)

Information to candidates:

Name of patient: Ms Ravenhill

You have been tasked to speak to Mr Ravenhill, the father of Rebecca Ravenhill. Rebecca's GP has referred her to the mental health service as she has low weight. In addition, her routine medical screen has highlighted no significant electrolyte abnormalities. Mr Ravenhill knows that his daughter has been dieting for some time. He is apprehensive about his daughter's condition and hopes to speak to someone from the mental health service about her condition. He hopes she could be sectioned under the Mental Health Act for mandatory treatment.

Task: Please speak to the father, Mr Ravenhill, and address all his concerns and expectations.

Outline of station:

You are Mr Ravenhill, the father of Rebecca Ravenhill. Rebecca is your only daughter, and you have been extremely concerned about her condition. You know that she has been dieting over the past few months. You decided she needed help and brought her to the GP two days ago. The GP has referred her over to the mental health services. You are hoping that some professional could help your daughter with her condition. You understand that there is a Mental Health Act and hope the professional could apply it to treating your daughter. You are at a loss about how best to help Rebecca. You are curious whether you could force-feed her. You wish to know more about the other treatment methods. In addition, you hope to be able to clarify with the mental health professional the criteria for admission. You are very anxious about your daughter as you have been her main caregiver since you divorced your wife ten years ago.

CASC Construct Table:

The CASC Construct Table is formatted such that candidates would be able to cover adequately both the range and depth of the assessment required in this station.

DOI: 10.1201/9781003313113-91

Starting off: "Hello, I am Dr Melvyn, one of the psychiatrists from the mental health unit. I understand that you have some concerns about your daughter. Could we have a chat?"			
Address expectations and concerns	I understand that you have been having some concerns with regard to your daughter's condition. I understand that she has been dieting over the past few months. Could you tell me more?	I understand you're deeply concerned about your daughter's condition. Regarding your concern about whether we could section your daughter for treatment, As we need to respect her personal rights, I'm sorry to tell you that we can't section her. There are other circumstances to which we might consider the utilization of the Mental Health Act, such as when the individual is actively suicidal. In some situations, she might lack the mental capacity to make decisions about her treatment options, and we could consider sectioning her.	I hear your concerns about your daughter's current weight. We need to commence re-feeding slowly, gradually. Forced feeding might be counter-therapeutic, and she might develop other complications.
Clarify the criteria for admission	We will consider recommending your daughter for a course of inpatient treatment if she has one of the following features:	The persistent decline in oral intake or rapid decline in the weight of more than 1 kg per week/Presence of heart rate abnormalities or blood pressure abnormalities/ Having low body temperature.	Severe electrolyte imbalance/worsening of an underlying psychiatric disorder or the failure of outpatient treatment.

Explain treatment options	There are various treatment strategies that we could adopt to help your daughter. A multidisciplinary team will work with her when she is admitted to the inpatient unit. As part of the treatment programme, we will focus on her medical needs and address any underlying psychological issues.	Weight restoration— Whilst she is an inpatient, we aim for a weight gain of 0.5–1 kg per week.	Feeding—We will work with a dietician prior to the initiation of feeding. If she does not gain the weight described, we will consider meal supervision or the administration of high-caloric feeds/fluids.
Explain management plans	Psychotherapy—There are various forms of psychotherapy that might be beneficial for patients. Examples of such psychotherapy include cognitive analytic therapy, cognitive behavioural therapy, interpersonal therapy, focal dynamic therapy, and family interventions. The main objectives of these therapies are to psycho-educate her on her condition, help her gain acceptance of her own body, and help her deal with her emotions and needs.	For inpatients, we usually recommend that outpatient psychological treatment be also offered on discharge, and we recommend a total duration of therapy to be around 12 months.	Pharmacotherapy— Medication is not used as the sole or primary treatment for the condition. Do you have any other questions for me? Thanks for sharing your concerns with me, and I do hope that I have addressed them accordingly.

Common pitfalls:

a. Failure to cover the range and depth of the information required for this station.
b. Failure to explain adequately the mechanism behind re-feeding syndrome and the range of electrolyte disturbances that result from it.
c. Failure correctly to advise on the rate of healthy caloric increase and weight gain in management.

Information to candidates:

Name of patient: Sarah Tewari

You have been tasked to speak to Laura, a community practice nurse who has been following up on one of the outpatients, Sarah Tewari. During the last home visit, she noted that Sarah's mother has insisted on forcing her child (Sarah) to binge-eat. Laura shared that Sarah has gained 2 kg over the past week. During one of her routine visitations to the local GP, it was discovered that there were several abnormalities in her blood test for Sarah. Laura is at a loss as to how best to help Sarah and hope you will be able to help her.

Task: Please speak to Laura, the community practice nurse who has been following up on the care of Sarah, and address all her concerns and expectations.

Outline of station:

You are Laura, the community practice nurse who has been following up on an outpatient named Sarah Tewari. You have known Sarah since her last hospitalization for her eating disorder issue one year ago. You note that her mother has been force-feeding Sarah, as her mother is quite upset with her daughter for constantly restricting her diet. You are aware that, in one week, Sarah has gained a total of 2 kg. During one of her routine follow-up check-ups with the local GP, it was discovered that Sarah had several blood abnormalities. You are very concerned about Sarah and wonder if she could be suffering from re-feeding syndrome. You wish to know more about this syndrome and how best to help Sarah with her condition.

CASC Construct Table:

The CASC Construct Table is formatted such that candidates would be able to cover adequately both the range and depth of the assessment required in this station.

DOI: 10.1201/9781003313113-92

Starting off: "Hello, I am Dr Melvyn, one of the psychiatrists from the mental health unit. I understand that you have been following up on Sarah Tewari. Could we have a chat about her condition?"			
Explore concerns	I understand you wanted to meet up with me as you have concerns about Sarah's condition. Could you tell me more?	You mentioned that she had gained weight rapidly over the past week. Could you share more with me? Does Sarah have any bodily symptoms of concern?	I also understand that she had some blood tests done with her local GP. Could you tell me more about the results of those tests? Could you share with me when Sarah was first diagnosed with an eating disorder? Did she require any previous inpatient hospitalization? How long have you been following up on her condition in the outpatient?
Explain the likely diagnosis of re-feeding syndrome	Thanks for sharing your concerns with me. It seemed that Sarah might have developed a condition known as re-feeding syndrome. Have you heard about it before?	Could I explain more about re-feeding syndrome? This is a condition in which individuals, usually those with eating disorders, are receiving additional calories too fast.	A variety of chemical imbalances and changes in the body usually characterizes it. Hence, this explains the abnormal blood results that Sarah has now. When additional calories are introduced into the body too rapidly, what happens is that the body would have to switch from fat metabolism over to carbohydrate metabolism. When this happens, it is commonly associated with a shift in the electrolyte and fluid balances. Hence, electrolytes such as potassium, magnesium, and phosphates are affected, and this would in turn cause a variety of clinical signs and symptoms.
Explain the signs and symptoms of re-feeding syndrome	There are a variety of signs and symptoms that patients might have when they develop the re-feeding syndrome. In Sarah's case, she has swelling of her hands and legs.	Other symptoms might include constipation, vomiting, diarrhoea, generalized lethargy, and abnormal heart rhythm.	Some patients might also develop seizures because of the re-feeding syndrome. In severe cases, they might also suffer from cardiac/ heart failure.

(Continued)

(Continued)

Explain management plans	I need your help to arrange a consultation with Sarah. If we are certain that she has the re-feeding syndrome, she cannot be managed as an outpatient.	I would need her to be admitted to the hospital for further inpatient treatment and stabilization.	We need to correct the electrolytes abnormalities and consider careful re-feeding with the help of our dietician and multidisciplinary team members. Do you have any other questions for me?

Common pitfalls:

a. Failure to cover the range and depth of the information required for this station.

b. Failure adequately to explain the mechanism behind re-feeding syndrome and the range of electrolyte disturbances that results from it.

c. Failure correctly to advise on the rate of healthy caloric increase and weight gain in management.

TOPIC VIII

PERSONALITY DISORDER

Information to candidates:

Name of patient: Ms Simmons

Ms Simmons, a 25-year-old female, has been admitted to the emergency services following her attempt to overdose on medication. This has been her third visit to the emergency services within the past month. The medical team is concerned about her recurrent overdoses and requested the on-call psychiatrist to speak to her to determine if she has any mental health issues. You are the on-call core trainee-3, and your consultant has requested that you assess the patient first.

Task: Please speak to Ms Simmons and obtain a complete history from her. Please get sufficient history in order to formulate a clinical diagnosis.

Outline of station:

You are Ms Simmons, and you have been transferred to the accident and emergency department following an attempt to overdose again. This is your third episode of overdosing this month. You have been having stressors mainly from your relationship difficulties. You have had a history of short and intense relationships. You feel abandoned and unloved in between relationships. You cut yourself or overdose at times to cope with the stressors arising from the relationships. There have also been times to when you have done impulsive acts. You are only willing to disclose more if the interviewer is nice and empathetic in questioning.

CASC Construct Table:

The CASC Construct Table is formatted such that candidates would be able to cover adequately both the range and depth of the assessment required in this station.

DOI: 10.1201/9781003313113-93

Starting off: "Hello, I am Dr Melvyn, one of the psychiatrists from the mental health unit. I understand that you have just been admitted to the emergency department. Could we have a chat?"			
Rapport building and history of presenting complaint and explore borderline traits—self-harm attempts	I received some information from the medical doctors. My understanding is that you have been admitted to the emergency department following an overdose. Am I right? I'm sorry to learn of that and understand that it must have been quite difficult for you.	Could you tell me more about what happened? Was there anything bothering you prior to the attempt?	Is this the first time that it has occurred? When did something similar happen? How recent was that? You mentioned that you have previously overdosed on medication before. Have you done anything else? You mentioned that you have cut yourself previously? How frequently was that? What do you use to cut? What was running through your mind when you cut yourself? Were you having thoughts of ending your life, or were you cutting yourself to release the stress and tension within?
Explore borderline traits—relationships	It seemed to me that your relationship issue was the main stressor that led to you having an overdose. I will be asking you a series of questions to understand you better and ascertain how best we could help you. How would you describe yourself as a person?	How do you usually cope when your relationship does not turn out well? How do you feel when your relationships end? Have you ever felt that you have been abandoned, especially so in between relationships?	How many relationships have you had now? How long does each relationship last for you?
Explore borderline traits—identity disturbances and impulsiveness	Could you tell me how you feel about yourself and your future?	Some people do tell me that they have this feeling of chronic emptiness. Have you have had such feelings and experiences before?	How would you describe yourself? Do you think you are very impulsive?

(Continued)

(Continued)

Explore borderline traits—affective instability	How has your mood been?	Do you find that there is much fluctuation in your mood? Have there been periods in which you experience intense anger or irritability?	What do others say about your mood?
Explore quasi-psychotic symptoms	With all these stressors that you have been enduring, has there been a time in which you have had unusual experiences?	I mean hearing voices or seeing things that are not there?	Could you tell me more?
Explore idealization and devaluation	Do you tend to rate people as either very good or very bad?	Do you tend to separate the good and bad people (splitting)?	
Other associated histories	Have you had any other mental health problems? Have there been episodes in which you restrict your weight or go on binges?	Have you used substances like alcohol or drugs to cope with your emotions?	Have there been any issues in your childhood? Do you recall any previous traumatic experiences? Have you been experiencing nightmares and flashbacks of the previous traumatic incident?

Common pitfall:

a. Failure to cover the range and depth of the information required for this station.

**If the patient mentions that she has been self-cutting, it would be worthwhile to offer to look at the cuts. This demonstrates empathy on your part and allows you to assess for the severity of the cuts and possible complications (e.g. infection or abscess).

TOPIC IX
WOMEN'S MENTAL HEALTH AND PERINATAL PSYCHIATRY

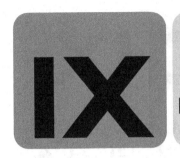

Information to candidates:

Name of patient: Ms Tatton

You have been tasked to speak to Ms Tatton, who is a 26-year-old female. She has just given birth to her child four weeks ago. Her partner noted that she has been increasingly emotional and tearful lately and has not been able to care for her child. He is very concerned about her condition and has brought her initially to the GP. The GP has referred her over to the mental health service.

Task: Please speak to Ms Tatton to elicit further history with regards to her condition and perform a risk assessment.

Outline of station:

You are Ms Tatton, and you gave birth to your child four weeks ago. This is your first child after an unplanned pregnancy. There are no problems during the pregnancy, and your relationship with your partner has been good. You find that you have become more emotional recently. You have not much interest in caring for your child. You tend to find yourself lethargic in the day. You worry that your child is lacking good care due to your lack of competency in taking care of him. You do not have any abnormal ideas about your child. You have had passive thoughts of suicide but have not planned anything concrete thus far.

CASC Construct Table:

The CASC Construct Table is formatted such that candidates would be able to cover adequately both the range and depth of the assessment required in this station.

DOI: 10.1201/9781003313113-94

Starting off: "Hello, I am Dr Melvyn, one of the psychiatrists from the mental health unit. I received a referral letter from your GP. Could we have a chat?"			
Presenting history	I understand that things have been difficult for you since you gave birth to your child. Could you tell me more?	I'm sorry to hear how you have been. How long have you been feeling this way for?	
Elicit risk factors	Have you have had similar episodes previously? Have you seen a psychiatrist before? Is there anyone in your family who has a history of any mental health illness?	Could you tell me more about your pregnancy? Is this a planned pregnancy? Is this the first time you have had a child? How were things when you had your baby? Was the antenatal checkup normal?	How was the delivery of your child? Were there any complications? Did your baby need extensive stay in the hospital after delivery? How is your relationship with your partner? Has he been supportive? Could you tell me what's your baby's name? Have you been able to bond with and care for your baby? Do you breast-feed your baby? Is there anyone else to help you with the care for your baby?
Assessment for depressive symptoms	You mentioned that you have been more emotional since your child's birth. How long has this been? Does your mood vary within the course of the day? Do you find yourself losing interest in things that you used to enjoy?	How have your energy levels been? Have there been any difficulties with your sleep? Can you tell me more? Do you have difficulties falling asleep, or do you have difficulties staying asleep?	How has your appetite been? Have you had things that you feel guilty about?
Assessment for psychotic symptoms	I understand that this has been a very difficult time for you.	Sometimes, when people undergo difficult situations in life, they have unusual experiences, such as hearing voices or seeing things that are not there. Have you have had these experiences?	Have you ever felt that someone out there is trying to do something to harm you or your baby? How certain are you about this? Do you feel that your thoughts are being interfered with? Do you feel that your emotions and actions are no longer under your control?

(Continued)

(Continued)

Risk assessment	Have you ever had thoughts that life is not worth living? Have you have had any thoughts of ending your life? Have you made any plans? Have you written any last notes to your loved ones?	What do you think would keep you from thinking about harming yourself?	Have you ever felt so low in mood that you have had thoughts about harming your baby? Could you tell me more about your plans (if any)?

Common pitfall:

a. Failure to cover the range and depth of the information required for this station.

**It is helpful if you ask for the name of the baby early at the start of the interview. This may make the interview more personal and help the patient to open up.

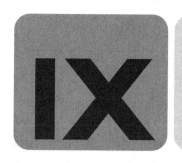

Information to candidates:

Name of patient: Mrs Tatton

You have been tasked to speak to Mrs Tatton, who is a 26-year-old female. She just gave birth to her child two weeks ago. Her husband noted that she has been increasingly emotional and tearful lately and has not been able to care for her child. Apart from her low mood, she has expressed concerns that her child might be harmed by a devil. Her GP has referred Mrs Tatton to the mental health services for an assessment today.

Task: Please speak to Mrs Tatton to elicit further history with regard to her condition and perform a risk assessment.

Outline of station:

You are Mrs Tatton, and you have given birth to your child two weeks ago. This is your first child after an unplanned pregnancy. There are no problems during the pregnancy and your relationship with your husband has been good. You find that you have become more emotional recently. You worry very much that a devil is out to harm your baby. You have heard voices telling you that you must keep your baby safe from the devil.

CASC Construct Table:

The CASC Construct Table is formatted such that candidates would be able to cover adequately both the range and depth of the assessment required in this station.

DOI: 10.1201/9781003313113-95

Starting off: "Hello, I am Dr Melvyn, one of the psychiatrists from the mental health unit. I received a referral letter from your GP. Could we have a chat?"			
Presenting history	I understand that things have been difficult for you since you gave birth to your child. Could you tell me more?	I'm sorry to hear how you have been. How long have you been feeling this way for?	
Elicit risk factors	Have you have had similar episodes previously? Have you seen a psychiatrist before? Is there anyone in your family with a history of mental health illness?	Could you tell me more about your pregnancy? Is this a planned pregnancy? Is this your first child? How were things when you were having your baby? Was the antenatal checkup normal?	How was the delivery of your child? Were there any complications? Did your baby need extensive stay in the hospital after delivery? How is your relationship with your husband? Has he been supportive? Could you tell me what's your baby's name? Have you been able to bond with and care for your baby? Do you breast-feed your baby? Is there anyone else to help you with the care for your baby?
Assessment for psychotic symptoms	I understand that it has been a very difficult time for you. Have you ever worried that someone wants to harm you and your baby? Could you tell me more? How certain are you that there is indeed someone who wants to do this? Is there any alternative explanation for this?	Are you worried that there is something wrong with your baby? If so, could you tell me more? Other symptoms: Any mood swings? Have there been times when you are confused about the time, place and person?	Have you heard voices after delivery? Could you tell me more? If so, did the voices ever give you any instructions, such as telling you to harm your baby? Do you feel in control of your thoughts? Or do you feel that your thoughts are being interfered with? Do you feel as if someone else could control the way you feel and the way you think and act?

Risk assessment	Have you ever had thoughts that life is not worth living? Have you had any thoughts of ending your life? Have you made any plans? Have you written any last notes to your loved ones?	What do you think would keep you from thinking about harming yourself? Any neglect of your baby's physical needs? Any physical abuse?	Have you ever felt so low in mood that you have had thoughts about harming your baby? Could you tell me more about your plans (if any)? What do you think will stop you from doing anything to your child? Where is the baby now? Is there anyone helping to take care of your baby?

Common pitfall:

a. Failure to cover the range and depth of the information required for this station.

**It is important to assess for orientation and signs of confusion in this patient as they are major signs of postpartum psychosis.

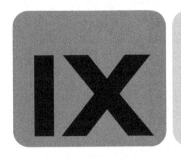

STATION 96 POSTNATAL PSYCHOSIS (PATIENT MANAGEMENT)

Information to candidates:

Name of patient: Mrs Tatton

You have previously been tasked to speak to Mrs Tatton, a 26-year-old female. She has just given birth to her child two weeks ago. Her husband noted that she has been increasingly emotional and tearful lately and has not been able to care for her child. Apart from her low mood, she has expressed concerns that a devil might harm her child. Her GP has referred Mrs Tatton to mental health services for an assessment today. She has since been assessed, and her husband is here, wishing to understand more about her condition and the wellbeing of his child. He wishes to know more about the plans the team has for his wife and child.

Task: Please speak to Mr Tatton, the husband of Mrs Tatton, and address all his concerns and expectations.

Outline of station:

You are Mr Tatton, the husband of Mrs Tatton, and you are highly concerned about her condition. You understand that the psychiatrist has seen your wife, and you wish to know more about the assessment. You want to know what condition your wife is suffering from. You wonder whether she might be having postpartum blues or postpartum depression. You hope that the team could help your wife with her condition. If the team suggests the commencement of any medication, you must appear to be very concerned with the side effects of the medication on your child as you know that your wife has been breast-feeding. You wonder whether there are any other alternatives to medication. You want to ensure the safety of both your wife and your child, and you wish to know from the team how best they could help ensure the safety.

CASC Construct Table:

The CASC Construct Table is formatted such that candidates would be able to cover adequately both the range and depth of the assessment required in this station.

DOI: 10.1201/9781003313113-96

Starting off: "Hello, I am Dr Melvyn, one of the psychiatrists from the mental health unit. I understand that you have some concerns about your wife's condition. Could we have a chat?"			
Clarification about diagnosis	I understand that you are very concerned about your wife's condition. We have seen your wife and have done an assessment. Can I share with you more about our assessment?	We feel that your wife might be suffering from a condition known as postpartum psychosis. Have you heard of this condition before?	This is a condition that usually commences abruptly two weeks after delivery. The patient usually has some affective features and unusual experiences such as delusions or hallucinations. They might feel that others are out to harm them or their child, or they might also hear voices. Do you know whether your wife has an existing mental health condition? If she does have, and especially if it is bipolar disorder, she is more predisposed towards this condition.
Explain management plans	I understand that you must be finding it tough to come to terms with the condition that your wife is having currently. Please let me reassure you that this is a condition that is highly treatable. We like to do our best to help your wife with her condition. Can I tell you more about how best we could offer your wife assistance with her condition?	One of the concerns that we have lies largely with the safety of her and your child. We would recommend admitting her to the mother and baby unit for further treatment and stabilization. The nursing staff in the unit would be able to monitor her condition, and we could also help her through the commencement of certain medication.	We would like to commence an antipsychotic medication for your wife. If medications do not help your wife, one other alternative that we could consider is the administration of electro-convulsive therapy (ECT). Have you heard about this form of therapy before? Can I take some time to explain more about the therapy to you? Apart from medication, we will also provide supportive counselling to help your wife with her condition. We will work closely with a multidisciplinary team consisting of a social worker and even an obstetrician to help your wife.

(Continued)

(Continued)

Explain potential complications if the patient is not treated	One of our concerns is that if your partner is not stabilized and treated, she might risk harming herself and her child.	Also, given her symptoms, she is not likely to be able to care for your child.	This will affect the parent-child bonding and would be detrimental to your child in the longer term. Studies have shown that it might result in emotional problems in the child.
Address concerns and expectations	I hope that I have managed to address all your concerns and expectations. Do you have any questions for me?	I hear that you are very concerned about the commencement of medication given that wife is breast-feeding. Please let me reassure you that we take this into consideration and will start her on a medication safe for use even if she is breast-feeding.	I also hear that you are very concerned about the usage of ECT for the treatment of your wife's condition. ECT has been demonstrated to be a safe and effective treatment for patients who are not responding to medication.

Common pitfall:

a. Failure to cover the range and depth of the information required for this station.

TOPIC X

CONSULTATION-LIAISON PSYCHIATRY

Information to candidates:

Name of patient: Mr Whitfield

You have been tasked to see Mr Whitfield, a 54-year-old gentleman who has just undergone hip surgery following a fall whilst he was intoxicated. His last drink, according to his daughter, was three days ago. He was noted to be very distressed and agitated in the ward and vocalized that he was having visual and auditory hallucinations. He has been threatening to leave the ward premises as well as he does not feel that the environment is safe. Your consultant, Dr Thomson, has heard about this patient and wishes to discuss the case with you.

Task: Please speak to Dr Thomson, your consultant on call, and discuss more about the case with him. Please summarize your findings and discuss a sound management approach for Mr Whitfield.

Outline of station:

You are Dr Thomson, the on-call consultant, and you have heard about this case as the nursing manager of the surgery ward has called you. You are aware that your core trainee has assessed the patient, and you hope that your core trainee can provide you with a summary of his assessment. You want to discuss with the trainee the differential diagnosis of the case and the most likely diagnosis given the clinical features. You would also like to discuss with the core trainee more about the specific management for the patient.

CASC Construct Table:

The CASC Construct Table is formatted such that candidates would be able to cover adequately both the range and depth of the assessment required in this station.

DOI: 10.1201/9781003313113-97

Starting off: "Hello, I am Melvyn, one of the core trainees. Could I discuss a case with you?"			
Brief formulation of current assessment	I have seen Mr Whitfield, who is a 54-year-old gentleman referred from the general surgery unit. My understanding is that he has been admitted following a recent fall and has just undergone an operation. I understand that he sustained the fall whilst he was intoxicated with alcohol around three days ago.	I have seen the patient; he is currently confused and not orientated to time, place, or person. He does have episodes of agitation, and it is quite hard for the nursing staff to manage him in the ward. He has been reporting both visual and auditory hallucinations.	He seemed quite distressed by the visual hallucinations he is experiencing. He does not find it safe to be in the ward and has been requesting for the team to consider discharging him.
Likely diagnosis and differential diagnosis	Given that he has the presence of altered consciousness, visual and auditory hallucinations, and considering that his last drink was three days ago, the most likely clinical diagnosis now is delirium tremens.	I have obtained a collaborative history from his daughter that suggest that he is alcohol dependent, and his last drink was around three days ago. He previously used a combination of beer and hard liquor.	I would like to consider other differential diagnoses as well. The blood investigations have been done and do not show an infective picture or sepsis now. The acute onset of the current presentation might not be typical for a patient with schizophrenia or other psychotic disorder.
Management—pharmacological	Delirium tremens is a medical emergency, and he needs immediate and close monitoring in a medical ward. Prior to the commencement of medication, I'd like to suggest that there should be more intensive monitoring of his vitals. There should be regular reorientation. He should also be nursed in a quiet room, with familiar nursing staff as well.	We need to urgently replace his thiamine by giving him intravenous thiamine replacement up to 500 mg three times a day. We could consider starting a reduced dose of lorazepam, based on his CIWA withdrawal scores. He should also be monitored closely for withdrawal seizures.	Given the agitated behaviour, antipsychotic medication such as haloperidol could be considered an adjunctive medication for agitation and aggression.

(Continued)

(Continued)

Management—psychological	We need to educate and explain to the family the symptom and the medical condition he is having now.	Educate and provide support to the nursing staff to alleviate anxiety. Consistent nursing care and reduction of excessive stimulation that may worsen his delirium.	Once he is out of delirium, we need to consider referring him to the addiction service for the counsellor to assess him and to provide motivational interviewing regarding his alcohol issues.

Common pitfall:

a. Failure to cover the range and depth of the information required for this station.

**It is important to mention the non-pharmacological methods before jumping into medication. Consider the approach of a multidisciplinary team. Highlight to the examiner that you can weigh the pros and cons of starting antipsychotic medication on a frail elderly patient.

STATION 98
CONVERSION DISORDER
(HISTORY TAKING)

Information to candidates:

Name of patient: Ms Griffin

Ms Tina Griffin is a 28-year-old female who has been admitted to the emergency services for acute onset of left-sided lower-limb weakness. Both the medical doctors and the neurologist have seen her, to which they do not think that she has any active medical illness. They understand from her mother that she has been through tremendous stress recently, and they feel that a psychiatric assessment is warranted.

Task: Please speak to Ms Griffin and obtain a relevant history to arrive at a diagnosis. Please perform an appropriate neurological examination.

Outline of station:

You are Ms Tina Griffin, and you have been brought into the emergency department following an acute onset of lower limb weakness. You were at your father's funeral when this happened. The significant stressor was that you were involved in a road traffic accident three days ago, in which you were the driver, and your father was killed. No one in the family has since blamed you for the accident, but you have felt very guilty for it as you could have been more cautious that day.

CASC Construct Table:

The CASC Construct Table is formatted such that candidates would be able to cover adequately both the range and depth of the assessment required in this station.

DOI: 10.1201/9781003313113-98

Starting off: "Hello, I am Dr Melvyn, one of the psychiatrists from the mental health unit. I received some information as to why you have been admitted. Could we have a chat?"			
History of current presenting complaint	I understand from the medical doctors that you have been admitted today. Can you tell me more about what happened this morning? You mentioned that you have been feeling weak in one of your legs. Which leg is this?	Do you remember what you did when you had this sudden numbness? Were there any other disturbing symptoms? Say, for example, did you have numbness or any tingling sensation? Any physical symptoms, for example, pain or deficits anywhere?	Have you experienced something like what you have experienced in the past?
Stressors precipitating onset of symptoms	Have there been any changes in life recently? Or have you been under any stress recently? Can you tell me more?	I'm sorry to hear that. You mentioned that you were at your father's wake when this happened.	Was your father's passing expected or unexpected? How do you feel about it?
Eliciting la belle indifference and checking for secondary gains	Since the time that you have been admitted, the medical doctors and the neurologists have checked upon you, and they have run some tests on you. Thus far, from my understanding, the test results are negative.	How do you feel about this sudden onset of weakness? Are you concerned about this? Are you relieved by the investigation findings? Do you believe what the doctors said?	How has your family members responded when they came to learn of the fact that you are having a weakness of your legs? Are they concerned? Have they made any alternative arrangements or accommodation for you?
Assess for comorbid psychiatric condition	Recently, how have you been feeling in your mood? Do you feel depressed or anxious? Are you still able to enjoy things that you used to enjoy previously?	How have your energy levels been like? What about your sleep and appetite?	Have you had any unusual experiences recently? Are things so troubling for you that you have entertained thoughts that life is not worth living?
Relevant personal and medical history	Have you been seen by a psychiatrist before? Does anyone in the family have any mental health conditions that I need to know of?	Do you have any other chronic medical conditions that we need to know of?	Do you take any drugs or substances to help you cope with the stress you are experiencing?
Neurological examination	Perform a neurological examination of the lower limbs		

Common pitfall:

a. Failure to cover the range and depth of the information required for this station.

**It is important to rule out another differential diagnoses, such as hypochondriasis, somatoform disorders, and malingering.

**Ask in a tactful manner how things have changed for the patient since developing the physical symptoms.

STATION 99 CONVERSION DISORDER (DISCUSSION OF MANAGEMENT PLANS)

Information to candidates:

Name of patient: Ms Griffin

Ms Tina Griffin is a 28-year-old female who has been admitted to the emergency services for acute onset of left-sided lower-limb weakness. Both the medical doctors and the neurologist have seen her, to which they do not think that she has any active medical illness. However, they understand from her mother that she has been through tremendous stress recently, and they feel that a psychiatric assessment would be warranted. You have previously spoken to Ms Griffin and have obtained a history to arrive at a diagnosis. You have also performed a neurological examination. Her mother is waiting to speak to you outside the consultation room.

Task: Please speak to Ms Griffin's mother, Mrs Anna Griffin, and explain to her more about her daughter's current condition. Please address all her concerns and expectations.

Outline of station:

You are Mrs Anna Griffin, the mother of Ms Tina Griffin. You are very concerned about your daughter's condition. You wish to know more about her diagnosis as you have understood from the medical doctors as well as the neurologists that there is nothing wrong with her with regards to the biochemical and the radiological investigations. You'd also like to know what the potential cause of her condition is and how you could manage her condition. You also wish to know how best you could help her with her current condition. Therefore, you tell the core trainee that you wish to know more about her condition.

CASC Construct Table:

The CASC Construct Table is formatted such that candidates would be able to cover adequately both the range and depth of the assessment required in this station.

DOI: 10.1201/9781003313113-99

Starting off: "Hello, I am Dr Melvyn, one of the psychiatrists from the mental health unit. I understand that you have some concerns about your daughter's condition. Could we have a chat about this?"			
Summarized findings	I understand that you have some concerns about your daughter's condition. I have assessed your daughter previously. Can I share my assessment with you?/Can I tell you more about her condition?	The medical team and the neurologists have done some blood works as well as imaging to find a cause for her sudden onset of lower limb weakness. I'm glad to inform you that, thus far, those findings are negative.	I understand from Tina that she has been under tremendous stress recently. I'm sorry to learn of the family situation recently. We have also done a complete neurological examination during our interview as well.
Explain diagnosis and causes	I understand that you are concerned about the diagnosis for your daughter. We feel that your daughter has a condition known as conversion disorder. Have you heard about this before?	In essence, there is a close interrelationship between our body and our mind. Hence, if one is affected, so is the other. For example, if you have experienced a lot of stress at work, it is not uncommon for you to have a physical symptom such as headache. In Tina's case, it seemed like the tremendous stress she has experienced has been converted into a physical symptom, which in her case would be the weakness of her lower limb.	Do you have any questions for me? The stress that she is experiencing is very real. However, this condition is usually temporary and would gradually improve with time. The stressor that causes this disorder are usually that of tremendous traumatic events, insolvable problems, and problematic relationships.
Explain management—pharmacological	There is a range of ways in which we could offer to help Tina with her current condition. As all the relevant investigations have been done and are negative, there is no further need to conduct any other investigations.	We would advise that she come back regularly, and we could monitor her mood. If her mood is low or she develops other psychiatric illnesses, we could treat them accordingly with medication.	Some patients do experience changes in their mood and might become depressed. In those circumstances, medication such as antidepressants is indicated.

(Continued)

(Continued)

Explain management—psychological	Apart from medication, there are other modalities of therapy that have been shown to be helpful.	Such therapies might include that of talking therapies such as cognitive behavioural therapy (CBT). Have you heard of this before?	The family is advised to avoid reinforcing Tina's weakness/inability to do things.
Address concerns and expectations	I understand that I have shared quite a lot of information. Do you have any questions for me?	I totally understand how concerned you are with regards to her condition. As her mother, I think the most important thing for you to do is to acknowledge that she has a real problem—she is dealing with a tremendous stressor. Your support would be important for her.	With regards to the prognosis of the condition, over time, people do recover well from the condition. I like to offer you some leaflets from the Royal College of Psychiatrists for you to have a better understanding of her condition.

Common pitfall:

a. Failure to cover the range and depth of the information required for this station.

STATION 100
HEALTH ANXIETY
DISORDER
(HISTORY TAKING)

Information to candidates:

Name of patient: Mr O'Connor

You have been tasked to speak to Mr O'Connor, a 35-year-old gentleman who has been referred by the neurologist. He has been referred to multiple neurologists previously for his headache. He has done multiple investigations, which to date all have been normal.

Task: Please speak to Mr O'Connor to obtain more history with regards to his symptoms. Please assess adequately to formulate a diagnosis.

Outline of station:

You are Mr O'Connor. You have been having persistent headache for the past couple of months. Several neurologists have seen you, and they have done basic blood works for you as well as radiological imaging scans. You have been told that there is nothing abnormal, but that only brings you temporary reassurance. You recently sought a consultation with another neurologist, who has decided to refer you to see a psychiatrist. You have been told that your headaches might be stress-induced and, hence, the referral.

CASC Construct Table:

The CASC Construct Table is formatted such that candidates would be able to cover adequately both the range and depth of the assessment required in this station.

DOI: 10.1201/9781003313113-100

Starting off: "Hello, I am Dr Melvyn, one of the psychiatrists from the mental health unit. I understand that your neurologist has referred you. Could we have a chat to understand your condition better?"			
History of presenting complaint	I understand from the memo from your neurologist that you have been troubled by headaches recently. Could you tell me more about your headaches? When did these headaches first start for you? How has the headache progressed since then?	Could you tell me whether there is anything that would make it better? Are there things that might make it worse than usual? Over this entire period, do you have other symptoms, such as weakness or nausea or vomiting?	I understand that you have previously consulted multiple neurologists. What have they told you? Have they done any blood tests or investigations? Did they share with you more about the results? Are you convinced by the results of the tests that you have undergone? How long did you feel reassured by the test results for before you needed to seek the advice of another doctor? Are you concerned that you might have an underlying brain issue? What brain condition do you think you have? What makes you feel that you are at risk with regards to this condition?
Impact on current life	Do you find yourself feeling very preoccupied that you might have an underlying brain condition? Have you been spending a lot of time reading up more about the various conditions? From whereabouts have you been getting your information from? Do you find yourself needing to get constant reassurance from your family members? (Or) What do your family members say to you regarding your condition?	How has this affected your life in general? Has this condition affected you in terms of your functioning? Are you able to do things like how you used to be able to? How is your relationship with your family members, loved ones, as well as with your friends?	Has this condition affected you in terms of your work at all? Are you able to perform like how you used to be able to at work?

Previous medical history, social and personal history	Can I check whether you have any past medical conditions I need to know? Do you have any long-term illnesses? Are you on any long-term medication?	What was your childhood like? Were you frequently sick? How did your family respond whenever you fell ill? Did they take you to the doctor every time for every single symptom?	Do you have any family members who have long-term conditions? Do you have family members who have been diagnosed with the condition that you have spoken about? Could you tell me more? When did you know that they have been suffering from such a condition? Was it just recently, over the past couple of months or so?
Other comorbidities	With all these going on and its impact on your life, how has your mood been like? Are you able to maintain interest in things that you used to enjoy doing?	How has your energy levels been like? Are you able to sleep? What about your appetite? How has your appetite been?	Sometimes when people are undergoing stressful experiences, they do report of unusual experiences. Have you ever had these experiences before? Do you find that with your current condition life is no longer worth living and that you might be better off dead?

Common pitfalls:

a. Failure to cover the range and depth of the information required for this station.
b. Failure to ascertain the degree of conviction of the thoughts adequately—whether they are overvalued ideas or delusional in intensity.

Information to candidates:

Name of patient: Mrs O'Connor

You have been tasked to speak to Mr O'Connor, a 35-year-old gentleman who has been referred by the neurologist. He has been referred to multiple neurologists previously for his headache. He has done multiple investigations, which to date all have been normal. You have previously spoken to Mr O'Connor to obtain a history of his presenting complaint as well as more information about his previous medical and personal history. You managed to arrive at a diagnosis at the end of the interview. Mrs O'Connor, his wife, is currently waiting outside the consultation room. She is very keen to speak to you to understand more about her husband's condition.

Task: Please speak to Mrs O'Connor with regards to her husband's condition. You are expected to discuss more about his diagnosis as well as the management options for her husband. Please address all her concerns as well as her expectations.

Outline of station:

You are Mrs O'Connor, the wife of Mr O'Connor. You understand that his neurologist has referred him over to see a psychiatrist. You are curious with regards to the reason for the referral. You hope that the core trainee could tell you more about your husband's diagnosis. In addition, you want to know what has caused him to be feeling this way. You are keen to learn more about the management options for your husband as you are keen for him to get better as soon as possible. You know that your husband needs you to be there to render him support emotionally most of the time. You wonder what else you could do to help your husband to get well sooner.

CASC Construct Table:

The CASC Construct Table is formatted such that candidates would be able to cover adequately both the range and depth of the assessment required in this station.

DOI: 10.1201/9781003313113-101

Starting off: "Hello, I am Dr Melvyn, one of the psychiatrists from the mental health unit. I understand that you have some concerns about your husband's condition. I have seen him. Could we have a chat about his condition?"

Establishing rapport and discussing diagnosis	I'm sorry to hear that you have been through quite a difficult time. It must be very tough for you in the past few months. I received information about the neurologists that he has been seeing that his blood tests and brain scans have been normal. They do not feel that your husband has any neurological or medical condition now, given the findings of the results.	I have previously just spoken to your husband and have assessed him accordingly. It seemed to me that your husband has a condition known as health anxiety disorder or hypochondriasis. Have you heard of this condition before?	The condition that your husband has is actually a very common condition. For some people, they tend to believe or fear that they would have a medical condition, even though their results are normal. Hence, it is not uncommon for them to repeatedly see various doctors and request for more tests as they are doubtful about the results. In addition, they would constantly be preoccupied with their condition and very often would constantly seek out for more information. They also tend to need constant reassurances.
Explaining causes	There has not been an established cause identified for this particular disorder.	Sometimes, it might be a resultant effect of someone who is living in a family who is very health conscious.	At times, stress could also be a trigger for someone to have such a condition. Chemical imbalances, particularly with regards to a brain chemical called serotonin, might contribute to the condition as well.
Explain management—pharmacological	There are various ways to which we could help your husband. Medication might be one option to which we could consider.	The medications that we feel might benefit your husband are antidepressants.	Antidepressants help to regulate the amount of serotonin in the brain and would help with his symptoms.

(Continued)

(Continued)

Explain management— psychological	Apart from medication, another option to which we could consider is engaging your husband in psychotherapy or talking therapy, such as cognitive behavioural therapy. Have you heard of this before?	As the name implies, there are two components to cognitive behavioural therapy. There is the cognitive component as well as the behavioural component. The goals of cognitive therapy are aimed towards reattribution and developing alternative explanations of symptoms and concerns of serious illness. Cognitive restructuring can modify dysfunctional assumptions.	The goals of behavioural therapy are aimed towards self-monitoring of worries, negative thoughts, and illness-related behaviours. It also involves exposure and response prevention and reducing repeated reassurance-seeking behaviours. The therapist would also help your husband to cope with his worries by teaching him relaxation techniques.
Address concerns and expectations	I understand that it is very stressful for you when your husband requests further evaluation. Given that he has been through multiple tests and investigations, further investigations would not be warranted currently.	I understand that it is very distressing for you given that he is constantly seeking reassurances from you. The reason why he needs reassurance is that it helps to provide temporary relief from his anxiety. This acts as a reward for him, and he is more likely to seek further reassurances from you.	Hence, it might be important for you to recognize these and continue to support him in the best way you could. We would advise him to continue routinely to attend his follow-up appointments with the psychologist. In addition, he should be maintained on the medication at the moment.

Common pitfall:

   a. Failure to cover the range and depth of the information required for this station.

**For hypochondriasis, it is important in the management to mention that containment of the patient to only one or two specialists to ensure consistency in the care and to prevent doctor hopping to get more investigations done.

STATION 102
SOMATOFORM
PAIN DISORDER
(HISTORY TAKING)

Information to candidates:

Name of patient: Mr Huston

You have been tasked to speak to Mr Huston, a 30-year-old gentleman. He has a chronic history of back pain and has been previously seen by multiple pain specialists for his chronic pain. He has done all the necessary blood investigations as well as imaging investigations, all of which has been normal thus far. His pain specialist has referred him over to your service for further assessment.

Task: Please speak to Mr Huston and obtain more history of his pain symptoms to come to a diagnosis.

Outline of station:

You are Mr Huston, and you have a chronic history of back pain. You have visited multiple pain specialists and have undergone multiple investigations, to which all have been normal thus far. You are not sure why one of your pain specialists has decided to refer you to a psychiatrist. You do not feel that you have any mental health condition, and you are reluctant to engage initially. You will share more about your pain symptoms only if the psychiatrist is empathetic in questioning. The main stressor currently is that your wife is very eager to have children, but you are not keen to have children now.

CASC Construct Table:

The CASC Construct Table is formatted such that candidates would be able to cover adequately both the range and depth of the assessment required in this station.

Starting off: "Hello, I am Dr Melvyn, one of the psychiatrists from the mental health unit. I understand that your pain specialist has referred you to see us. Could we have a chat?"			
History of presenting complaint	I understand that you must be feeling frustrated for your pain specialist to refer you to our service, given that you believe that you do not have any mental health condition. However, I understand that you have been having this pain for quite some time, and clearly you have been quite distressed by it. I might be able to help you to cope with this stressor if only I could find out more about your symptoms. Would you be willing to share more about your symptoms with me?	I understand that this pain has been troubling you for quite some time. Could you tell me when it first started? How would you describe the pain that you first experienced? Was the pain localized to any areas of your body? How has the pain been since then? Has it been progressively worsening in nature? Can you tell me more about the pain currently?	Can you share with me whether there are any factors that could make the pain better? Can you share with me whether there are any factors that could make the pain worse? I understand that several specialists have seen you for your pain symptoms. Can you tell me whether they have done any specific investigations to look for the causes of your kind? Do you happen to know the outcomes of those tests? Given the findings of the tests, what do you think is the possible cause of your pain symptoms?
Aetiological factors precipitating pain symptoms	Sometimes, stressors in life might contribute to pain symptoms as well. Have there been any changes in life recently prior to the onset of the pain symptoms?	Have any problems with relationships at home (with your loved ones and your family members)? Have there been any difficulties or concerns with regards to your children?	Have there been any major stressors from work? (Or) How have you been coping with work? Do you have any financial concerns recently? Do you have other medical conditions that I need to know of? Are you told of your medical condition just recently?
Impact of current symptoms on life	I'm sorry to hear that this pain has been bothering you for so many months. Furthermore, I'm sorry to learn of the circumstances prior to the onset of your pain symptoms.	Has your current condition affected your lifestyle? (Or) Did your lifestyle change as a result of your current pain condition?	

Ruling out other psychiatric disorders	With all these going on, how has your mood been in the past month or so? Are you still able to enjoy things that you previously used to enjoy?	What about your energy levels? Do you feel lethargic easily? How has your sleep been? How has your appetite been? Do you have difficulties with concentration or attention?	Sometimes, when people are undergoing stressful circumstances, they do report of having some unusual experiences, such as hearing voices or seeing things that are not there. Does this sound like what you have experienced before? Have things been so stressful for you that you feel that life has no meaning? Have you contemplated of ending your life in view of your current problems? How have you coped with the problems so far? Do you use any substances such as alcohol or street drugs to help you cope with the symptoms?

Common pitfall:

a. Failure to cover the range and depth of the information required for this station.

**It is important to differentiate somatoform disorder (preoccupied with bodily symptoms) from health anxiety disorder (preoccupied with having a serious illness). Ask broadly for various physical symptoms from across different body systems, e.g. neurological, gastrointestinal, and genitourinary.

Information to candidates:

Name of patient: Mr Fordyce

You have been tasked to speak to Mr Fordyce. He was involved in a traumatic car accident about two years ago, in which he sustained a head injury and needed an operation for. Postoperatively, he recovered well and managed to gradually get back to his premorbid functioning. However, recently, his wife has noted that Mr Fordyce has been different in terms of his behaviour and personality. She is very concerned about the recent changes. She has brought him to the GP, who has in turn referred her to your service. She is here with him.

Task: Please speak to Mr Fordyce's wife and elicit a history of personality change. Please take sufficient history to come to a formulation.

Outline of station:

You are the wife of Mr Fordyce. You have been married to Mr Fordyce for five years. Two years ago, he was involved in a major car accident and sustained an injury to his head, which he needed surgery for. You were thankful that postoperatively, he managed to recover well. Your only concern currently is that it seemed that he has been different in terms of his behaviour and personality over the past few months. At times, he seemed to be quite disinhibited and would be overly familiar and make inappropriate remarks. Due to this, you have not attended church for a while as he made inappropriate remarks whilst in church. At times, you have noticed that he does appear to be more aggressive and irritable in this temper. His memory is not as good as how it used to be. He has not vocalized any other symptoms to you. You are concerned about his changes in personality and hope that someone could advise you the reasons for the changes in his behaviour.

CASC Construct Table:

The CASC Construct Table is formatted such that candidates would be able to cover adequately both the range and depth of the assessment required in this station.

DOI: 10.1201/9781003313113-103

Starting off: "Hello, I am Dr Melvyn, one of the psychiatrists from the mental health unit. I understand that your GP has referred your husband to see us. Could we have a chat about his problems?"			
History of presenting complaint	I understand that your GP has referred your husband, Mr Fordyce, for an assessment. I understand you have some concerns. Would you mind telling me more?	I'm sorry to learn how difficult things have been for you recently. Can you tell me when you first observed these changes? Was it immediately after the accident or just recently? How has things progressed since the time from which you first noticed till now? Have things been worsening?	Could you tell me more about the accident in which Mr Fordyce was involved? What injuries did he sustain? Did he lose consciousness at all? You mentioned that he needed to undergo a surgery. Could you tell me more about what surgery has been done? Did the neurologist or the surgeon follow up on his care? What have they said about his current condition?
Explore personality changes	Can you tell me more about your husband's personality prior to the recent accident? Can you tell me more with regards to how his personality has changed?	Does he seem to be more disinhibited? Has he done anything that is sexually inappropriate?	Does he seem to be more overfamiliar at times with strangers? Does he seem to be more impulsive in nature? Could you give me some examples?
Explore behavioural changes	Can you tell me more with regards to how his behaviour has changed?	Does he seem to be easily annoyed? Would he get frustrated easily? Does he appear to be sensitive to noise and light?	Has he been verbally aggressive at home? Has he been physically aggressive at home?
Explore judgement	How has his attention and concentration been?	Does he have any difficulties with making decisions?	What about his judgement?
Explore memory difficulties	How has his memory been? You mentioned that he has been having some difficulties in his memories.	Does he have any difficulties with his short-term memory? What about his long-term memory? Any problems with planning of activities? Does he have any problems with task shifting? Does he appear to be slow in his thinking at times?	Is he able to recognize people whom he has not seen for some time? Does he seem to be muddled up with the days and dates in a week? Does he have any difficulties with expenses and finances? Does he have any difficulties with finding the right words? Does he tend to repeat the words that he has already said? Is he still able to handle and manage himself? Does he need any form of assistance currently?

(Continued)

(Continued)

Exclude other psychiatric disorders	How has his mood been? Is he still able to have interest in things that he used to enjoy?	How is his energy level like? How has his sleep been? What about his appetite?	Has there been any other abnormal behaviours that you have noticed?
Risk assessment	Has he expressed any ideations of ending his life?	Has he expressed any ideations to hurt or harm anyone in particular?	

Common pitfall:

a. Failure to cover the range and depth of the information required for this station.

STATION 104
POST–MYOCARDIAL INFARCTION DEPRESSION (HISTORY TAKING)

Information to candidates:

Name of patient: Mr Silvers

You have been tasked to speak to Mr Silvers, a 55-year-old gentleman who has been recently admitted to the cardiac inpatient unit following a myocardial infarction. Since his discharge from the hospital, the cardiologist has linked him up with the cardiac rehabilitation programme. He has managed to participate in two sessions thus far but has been missing the scheduled sessions recently. In addition, he has mentioned to his GP that he has been feeling low in his mood recently. His GP has hence initiated a referral to the mental health service.

Task: Please speak to Mr Silvers and take a history with the aim of establishing a clinical diagnosis. Please also assess his current social circumstances and assess his current understanding with regards to his condition.

Outline of station:

You are Mr Silvers and you have just been admitted inpatient for a myocardial infarction. You have been treated, and your cardiologist has recommended that you participate in the cardiac rehabilitation programme after your discharge. You have managed to make it for two sessions thus far but have been missing the remaining sessions. You find that your mood has been low, and you do not have much interest to do things you used to enjoy. You do know the importance of participating in the programme and adhering to the recommendations of the cardiologist with regards to diet. Ever since your heart issue, you have not been able to get back to your normal work. You previously worked as a physical education teacher. Your wife is supportive, but recently she has also needed to work overtime, so there is no one at home. You have been feeling useless and helpless at home.

CASC Construct Table:

The CASC Construct Table is formatted such that candidates would be able to cover adequately both the range and depth of the assessment required in this station.

DOI: 10.1201/9781003313113-104

Starting off: "Hello, I am Dr Melvyn, one of the psychiatrists from the mental health unit. I understand that your GP has referred you to see us. Could we have a chat?"			
Elicit information about recent hospitalization and plans on discharge	I understand from the referral memo that you have recently been admitted inpatient following a heart attack. I'm sorry to learn of that. Could I understand more about your recent admission?	Could you tell me more about what happened prior to your admission to the cardiac unit? What were the symptoms you had that caused you to suspect that you have had a heart attack?	Could you tell me what treatment the cardiologist has given you so far? How has your recovery been? How long did you need to stay inpatient? Did the doctors prescribe any medication for you to take on a long-term basis on discharge? Did the doctors recommend that you take part in any specific programmes on discharge? Could you tell me more? Have you been going for the programmes on discharge?
Elicit core symptoms of depression	You mentioned that you have attended some of the sessions but recently have missed the scheduled sessions because you have been feeling low. How long have you been feeling low in your mood for? Does your mood vary across the time course of a day?	Are you still able to enjoy things that you used to be able to enjoy? How have your energy levels been like? How has your sleep been? What about your appetite? How has your attention and concentration been like?	Sometimes, patients do mention that they do experience unusual experiences when their mood is low. Have you ever had such experiences before? I'm sorry to learn that you have been through a very tough time. Do you feel that life is ever not worth living?
Elicit current stressors	Is there anything in particular that is a stressor for you ever since you were discharged?	How have things been at home? Have there been any relationship difficulties? Do your family members and loved ones understand your condition?	Did you used to work before this? Have you been able to get back to work since the heart attack? Did they make any special accommodation for you at work? Do you have any other concerns such as finances?

Elicit patient's understanding with regards to his condition	You mentioned that the cardiologist recommends that you take part in the cardiac rehabilitation programme. Did he tell you more about the programme?	Has the cardiologist given you any other advice about how best to manage your current condition? Did the cardiologist tell you the reasons as to why there is a need to modify some area of your current lifestyle?	It seems to me that your mood is low at the moment. We can help you with this. Do you think you will still be keen to continue on with the recommended programme if your mood is slightly better?

Common pitfall:

a. Failure to cover the range and depth of the information required for this station.

Information to candidates:

Name of patient: Mr Silvers

You have been tasked to speak to Mr Silvers, a 55-year-old gentleman who has been recently admitted to the cardiac inpatient unit following a myocardial infarction. Since his discharge from the hospital, the cardiologist has linked him up with the cardiac rehabilitation programme. He has managed to participate in two sessions thus far but has been missing the scheduled sessions recently. He has mentioned to his GP that he has been feeling low in his mood recently. His GP has hence initiated a referral to the mental health service. You have in the previous station spoken to the patient and elicited a history to come to a diagnosis. You have also explored his recent stressors and his motivation to engage in the cardio rehabilitation programme.

Task: Please speak to the consultant psychiatrist and discuss with the consultant the most appropriate management plan for this patient.

Outline of station:

You are the consultant psychiatrist, and you want to know more details with regards to the patient that the core trainee has just assessed. You wish to know the patient's understanding of his current condition, as well as his attitude towards his medical condition. You wish to discuss with the trainee the prevalence of depression amongst individuals with IHD as well as the mortality rates. You hope that the trainee has formulated a management plan in accordance with the guidelines and in consideration of the IHD history.

CASC Construct Table:

The CASC Construct Table is formatted such that candidates would be able to cover adequately both the range and depth of the assessment required in this station.

DOI: 10.1201/9781003313113-105

Starting off: "Hello, I am Melvyn. I have just spoken to and assessed Mr Silvers. Could I discuss the case with you?"

Summary of case	Mr Silvers is a 55-year-old gentleman who has been recently admitted for a myocardial infarction. He currently has low mood with reduced interest and poor engagement with his cardiac rehabilitation programme.	His ongoing stressors include that of him not being able to go back to work and function like what he used to be able to.	Clinically, he is depressed, and he fulfils the ICD-10 diagnostic criteria for depressive disorder. He does have an understanding as to why he needs to continue with the cardiac rehabilitation programme, and he is still motivated to engage if his mood symptoms are better sorted out. My current diagnosis for him is that of a post–myocardial infarction depressive disorder.
Prevalence and associated mortality rates	Based on my understanding, the prevalence of the depressive disorder in post–myocardial infarction patients is around 20%.	As compared to normal individuals, the mortality rate is enhanced, at a rate of two to six times higher.	
Management—pharmacological	With these in mind, I'd like to propose both pharmacological and non-pharmacological approaches to help him with his depressive disorder and to get him back into his cardiac rehabilitation programme.	With regards to medication, we need to take into consideration the recommendations of the SADHART trial. The trial proposed that sertraline is more suitable for patients post–myocardial infarction.	I would be cognizant not to start him with antidepressants such as the tricyclic antidepressants or venlafaxine, as tricyclic could cause irregular heart rhythms, and venlafaxine could cause an elevated blood pressure.

(Continued)

(Continued)

Management—non-pharmacological	In addition to medication, I'd like to refer the patient for psychological treatments, such as cognitive behavioural therapy (CBT) as well. Through CBT, he will learn behavioural and cognitive techniques to help him with his low mood.	In addition to psychological treatment, counselling services might also be beneficial for him, as they could educate him about lifestyle changes he needs to make. There is specific cardiac rehabilitation programme that could help structure an activity and nutrition plan to help with his recovery.	We could also refer him to get some support from social groups.
Management—others	I would liaise closely with the cardiologist and update the cardiologist about the treatment we have started for the patient.	Eventually, we hope that we could get the patient back on board the cardiac rehabilitation programme so that he could get back to his normal functioning in due course.	

Common pitfalls:

a. Failure to cover the range and depth of the information required for this station.
b. Failure to provide holistic management targeting depression and MI.

STATION 106 ANTIDEPRESSANT-INDUCED SEXUAL DYSFUNCTION (HISTORY TAKING)

Information to candidates:

Name of patient: Mr Mahdi

You have been tasked to speak to a 40-year-old male, Mr Mahdi. He has been recently diagnosed with depression and has been started on fluoxetine 20 mg by the mood disorder team. He has requested for an early review today, as he claimed that he has been experiencing some problems since the commencement of the antidepressant. He has been on the medication for the past six months.

Task: Please speak to him and explore more about his concerns regarding the antidepressant. Please try to obtain further history from him regarding his current concerns.

Outline of station:

You are Mr Mahdi, and you were diagnosed with depression approximately six months ago. The team has recommended that you be commenced on an antidepressant called fluoxetine. You have been compliant with this medication thus far. However, you have been concerned as the sexual side of your relationship appears to be affected as well. You thought that this might be due to your depression, but you personally feel that your mood symptoms have improved since the commencement of the medication. Prior to this, you did not have any difficulties with the sexual side of your relationship. You do not have any underlying medical conditions that might account for the current difficulties. You should appear to be initially reluctant to discuss this with the doctor. You will be willing to discuss more only if the doctor is empathetic.

CASC Construct Table:

The CASC Construct Table is formatted such that candidates would be able to cover adequately both the range and depth of the assessment required in this station.

DOI: 10.1201/9781003313113-106

Starting off: "Hello, I am Dr Melvyn. I hear that you wish to come off the antidepressant that we have recently started you on. Can we have a chat about it?"			
Explore the rationale for the commencement of antidepressant	I understand that we have started you on fluoxetine just recently. Can you tell me more about when it first started for you? Can I understand more about what happened back then that caused you to feel down? The onset of symptoms: Which came first—low mood or sexual dysfunction?	It has been some time since you have been on the antidepressant. Were there any initial difficulties with the medication? How has your mood been?	Do you feel that the medication has helped you? I understand that you wish to stop the medication. Can you please let me know why you wish to do so?
Explore current symptoms	I'm sorry to hear that you have been having difficulties with your relationship since you have been on the medication. How has your mood been? What score would you give your mood currently?	Are you able to enjoy things which you used to enjoy? Can you give me some examples? How have your energy levels been? How has your sleep been for you? Have there been any difficulties with your appetite?	Have you had thoughts that life is not worth living and that the future is hopeless? Have you ever had thoughts of ending your life? What are your plans forward? It's good to hear from you that your mood has been more stable since the commencement of the antidepressant.
Explore relationship difficulties	It is not uncommon for some individuals to experience some side effects from the medication. I'm sorry to hear that the medication has been causing you some issues with your relationship. In addition, this is something that we deal with on a regular basis, so please be assured that you can find a solution to help you with it.	I might need to speak to you and your partner about this. Would this be all right for you? I'm sorry that I might need to ask you some very personal questions. I understand that you have been having some relationship difficulties, in particular, with the sexual side of your relationship. Can you tell me more about your current difficulties?	Are there any problems with your interest in sex? Are there problems with you having an arousal or an erection? Are you able to perform and ejaculate during intimacy? Can you share with me more about how things were prior to the commencement of the antidepressant? In addition, have there been any other difficulties with your relationship with your partner?

Exclude other causative factors	Can I check whether you do have any medical problems that I need to know of? Are you on regular medication?	Can you tell me more about the control of your chronic conditions? How has your diabetes control been?	Since the onset of your depression, has it affected your relationship with your wife?
Explore and address patient's concerns	Thanks for sharing with me your concerns. Given the recent onset of your depression, I would recommend that you be kept on treatment for the next couple of months. I hear that you have some concerns about how the antidepressant might have an effect on the sexual side of your relationship.	Given that you have responded well to this medication, I strongly feel that you should be kept on the same medication. What we could do is to consider perhaps a drug holiday over the weekends and see if your symptoms could get better.	Alternatively, we could consider switching you to an alternative antidepressant, such as bupropion, that has a lesser impact on the sexual side of your relationship. Do you have any other questions for me? Would you mind I discuss further with your wife?

Common pitfall:

a. Failure to cover the range and depth of the information required for this station.

TOPIC XI

FORENSIC PSYCHIATRY

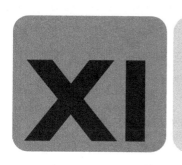

STATION 107
ASSAULT IN WARD
(PAIRED STATION A)

Information to candidates:

Name of patient: Mr Mayhew

You have been tasked to assess Mr Mayhew, a 40-year-old male. Mr Mayhew has been admitted two days ago for a relapse of his underlying psychiatric condition. This morning, he has assaulted one of the other patients. The nursing team is very concerned about his aggression and have requested for an immediate assessment.

Task: Please speak to Mr Mayhew and find out more information with regards to the assault this morning. Please also perform a mental state examination as well as a risk assessment.

Outline of station:

You are Mr Mayhew, and you have a history of schizophrenia. You have been admitted to the inpatient unit two days ago, and you are brought into the hospital by the assertive outreach team. You have not been compliant with your medication recently. You have been bothered by the increasing frequencies of the auditory hallucinations. You suspect that others on the ward might have plotted against you. This morning, the other patient stared at you, and you are convinced that he is the mastermind behind the plotting. You felt you needed to do something to stop others from troubling you. You do not think you are responsible for what happened this morning. You just did what was right to protect yourself.

CASC Construct Table:

The CASC Construct Table is formatted such that candidates would be able to cover adequately both the range and depth of the assessment required in this station.

DOI: 10.1201/9781003313113-107

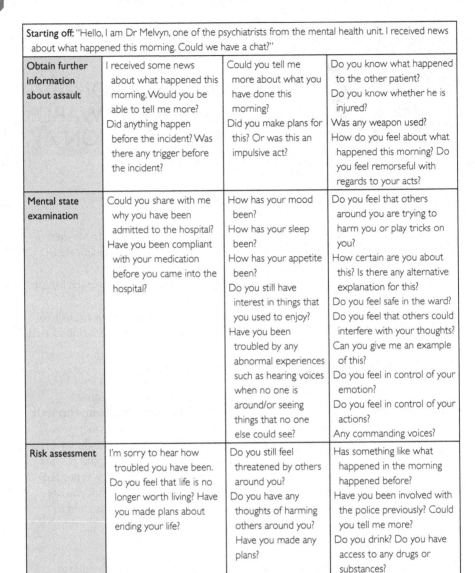

Starting off: "Hello, I am Dr Melvyn, one of the psychiatrists from the mental health unit. I received news about what happened this morning. Could we have a chat?"			
Obtain further information about assault	I received some news about what happened this morning. Would you be able to tell me more? Did anything happen before the incident? Was there any trigger before the incident?	Could you tell me more about what you have done this morning? Did you make plans for this? Or was this an impulsive act?	Do you know what happened to the other patient? Do you know whether he is injured? Was any weapon used? How do you feel about what happened this morning? Do you feel remorseful with regards to your acts?
Mental state examination	Could you share with me why you have been admitted to the hospital? Have you been compliant with your medication before you came into the hospital?	How has your mood been? How has your sleep been? How has your appetite been? Do you still have interest in things that you used to enjoy? Have you been troubled by any abnormal experiences such as hearing voices when no one is around/or seeing things that no one else could see?	Do you feel that others around you are trying to harm you or play tricks on you? How certain are you about this? Is there any alternative explanation for this? Do you feel safe in the ward? Do you feel that others could interfere with your thoughts? Can you give me an example of this? Do you feel in control of your emotion? Do you feel in control of your actions? Any commanding voices?
Risk assessment	I'm sorry to hear how troubled you have been. Do you feel that life is no longer worth living? Have you made plans about ending your life?	Do you still feel threatened by others around you? Do you have any thoughts of harming others around you? Have you made any plans?	Has something like what happened in the morning happened before? Have you been involved with the police previously? Could you tell me more? Do you drink? Do you have access to any drugs or substances? Do you feel that you are responsible for what happened this morning?

Common pitfall:

a. Failure to cover the range and depth of the information required for this station.

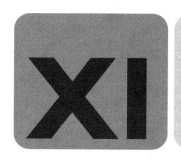

Information to candidates:

Name of patient: Mr Mayhew

You have been tasked previously to assess Mr Mayhew, a 40-year-old male. Mr Mayhew has been admitted two days ago for a relapse of his underlying psychiatric condition. This morning, he has assaulted one of the other patients. The nursing team is very concerned about his aggression and have requested for an immediate assessment. You have done the necessary assessment of the mental state of the patient, as well as a risk assessment. The ward manager, Mr DaSilva, has requested to speak to you regarding Mr Mayhew as he likes to know how the multidisciplinary team could help support and care for this patient.

Task: Please speak to Mr DaSilva and explain to him your assessments. Please formulate a joint management plan with him as the ward manager. Please address all his concerns and expectations.

Outline of station:

You are Mr DaSilva, the ward manager of the psychiatric ward. You are aware that Mr Mayhew, one of your patients, has assaulted another patient this morning. You are very concerned as you are worried that the victim's family would file a complaint. You hope to discuss the management plans with the core trainee. You wish to know about the patient's current mental state and risk assessment. You expect the core trainee to suggest some management plans to help contain the aggression of Mr Mayhew.

CASC Construct Table:

The CASC Construct Table is formatted such that candidates would be able to cover adequately both the range and depth of the assessment required in this station.

Starting off: "Hello, I am Dr Melvyn. I understand that you have some concerns about what happened this morning in the ward. Could we discuss how best to manage Mr Mayhew?"			
Explain mental state and risk assessment	I have seen the patient, and I hope to be able to answer the concerns that you have. I do understand that this is indeed a very difficult time for yourself and your colleagues in the ward.	When I interviewed him earlier, he shared with me that he assaulted the other patient as he felt that the other patient was attempting to harm him. He is convinced of this just by the way the other patient looked at him.	I understand that he has just been admitted to the ward around two days ago. It seemed to me that he is not very settled with his current medication regiment and is still quite paranoid and psychotic. Currently, he tells me that he no longer harbours any thoughts or plans to deal with any other patients or your staff. I understand from his records that he has no previous forensic history as well and has not abused any substances such as alcohol or drugs.
Discuss pharmacological management plans	Given that he is still quite unwell, we might need to consider increasing the dose of the antipsychotics medication that he is currently on.	In addition, we might want to consider using antipsychotics as per the rapid tranquilization protocol of the hospital. We could use sedating oral antipsychotics such as olanzapine or consider other intramuscular options such as intramuscular haloperidol or even intramuscular Ativan should he act out again.	We do need however to watch his vitals carefully following the administration of these medications. We should only use these medications if he is extremely agitated and cannot be managed by de-escalation or seclusion techniques.
Discuss alternatives to pharmacological management	There are other viable alternatives to medication. He might benefit from being more closely monitored and, ideally, if he could be constantly monitored by a staff that he is familiar with.	We could also house him in the seclusion room to allow him to settle if he is irritable or agitated.	The other alternative is to provide him with activities such as games to keep him engaged.

| Discuss forensic issues pertaining to fitness to plead | I understand the concerns that you have with regard to the incident this morning; in particular, with regard to whether the victim's family might file a complaint. | We might need to get our forensic colleagues to assess the patient if there are complaints made against the patient. | However, even though he has an existing mental health disorder, it does not negate the fact that he still needs to take responsibility for his actions and is still fit to be interviewed by the police should there be a complaint and there be further investigations. Do you have any other questions for me? |

Common pitfall:

a. Failure to cover the range and depth of the information required for this station.

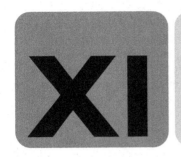

Information to candidates:

Name of patient: Ms Fields

You have been tasked to speak to a 17-year-old female, Ms Catherine Fields. She has been arrested by the police for arson and has been brought into the emergency department for an assessment. The police might consider charging her, but they hope that a psychiatric evaluation can be conducted first, as she seemed to be quite hysterical when she was remanded.

Task: Please speak to Ms Fields and elicit a history with regard to the arson that she has been involved in. Please obtain as much history as you can for you to formulate a diagnosis.

Outline of station:

You are Ms Catherine Fields, a 17-year-old female, and you have been arrested by the police for setting fire to the apartment that you are currently living in. This is not the first time you have set fire to your apartment. What happened today was that you chanced upon a television programme on BBC which showed how young children have been physically bullied by their caregivers. This reminded you of your past childhood experiences. You felt frustrated after watching the show and needed a channel to vent your frustration. You found a lighter in your room and made use of it to light up some papers in the wastepaper basket. You did not expect the fire to spread so quickly, and neither did you expect your neighbours to call upon the police. You realize that was wrong for you to do this. You have no previous mental health problems, and you did not use alcohol or any substances when you set your apartment on fire.

CASC Construct Table:

The CASC Construct Table is formatted such that candidates would be able to cover adequately both the range and depth of the assessment required in this station.

DOI: 10.1201/9781003313113-109

Starting off: "Hello, I am Dr Melvyn. I understand that the police have brought you in to our emergency services. I have only a limited understanding of what happened this morning. Would you mind sharing with me more?"			
Establish rapport and explore antecedents prior to the incident	I understand that it has been a difficult time for you.	Can you tell me what happened that caused you to be arrested by the police?	Are you able to tell me more? What happened before you started the fire?
Explore the fire-setting behaviour	Can you share with me more about how you started the fire?	Did you make any plans prior? Was it just out of impulse?	
Explore consequences of actions	Do you remember what happened after you started the fire?	Do you know who called upon the police? Did you think about the consequences—risk to self, others, and property?	Are you regretful of your actions?
Exclude comorbid psychiatric conditions	Thanks for sharing with me. Can I clarify—Is this the first time you have been involved in fire setting?	How did you feel before you set the fire? Were you feeling tensed up? How did you feel after that? Did you feel that there was a sudden release of tension? Were there times when you felt sexually aroused while setting the fire? Did you have the intention to end your life when you set the fire?	How has your mood been recently? Do you find that you still have an interest in things you used to enjoy? Has there been a time in which you had abnormal experiences? By that, I mean hearing things that are not there or seeing things that are not there?
Explore underlying triggers/past childhood issues	It seemed that what happened today reminded you of your past.	I understand that it might be difficult for you to share, but I'm hoping you could tell me if there were incidents in the past that were particularly significant, even up to today.	Have you been bullied before when you were much younger?
Rule out substance history	Did you use any alcohol prior to the recent incident?		

Common pitfall:
a. Failure to cover the range and depth of the information required for this station.

**The patient in this station may be difficult to engage. Thus, it is important for you to be empathetic and gently probe about the circumstances of the fire. Sometimes, if the patient refuses to talk, it may be helpful to go around the topic and ask about more neutral topics (e.g. personality) before going back to the pertinent issues. The patient's tone of voice may also be soft. Therefore, you may get permission to sit slightly closer to talk.

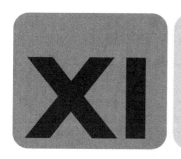

STATION 110
MORBID JEALOUSY
(HISTORY TAKING)

Information to candidates:

Name of patient: Mr Jenner

You have been tasked to speak to Mr Jenner. Mr Jenner was arrested this morning, as his wife called the police after he used a knife to threaten her. He has been suspicious about his wife's coming home late and has attributed it to her having an extramarital affair.

Task: Please speak to Mr Jenner and try to elicit as much history as possible to come to a diagnosis

Outline of station:

You are Mr Jenner and are upset that the police have detained you and have sent you over to a mental health service for an assessment. You should start off vocalizing your unhappiness at how the police have managed the situation and go on to mention more about your wife's problem. You have noticed that she has been coming home late these days. You went through her personal belongings a couple of days ago, and to your surprise, you found the name card of a male business partner. You firmly believe that she must be having an affair, which would explain why she has been coming home late and explain why she has not been interested in intimacy of late. You planned to make use of the knife today to threaten her into admitting her mistake. You do not have any plans to make use of the knife to hurt her. You use alcohol daily, but you do not use any other drugs. You do not have any previous forensic records of note.

CASC Construct Table:

The CASC Construct Table is formatted such that candidates would be able to cover adequately both the range and depth of the assessment required in this station.

DOI: 10.1201/9781003313113-110

Starting off: "Hello, I am Dr Melvyn. I understand that the police have brought you in to our emergency services. I have only a limited understanding of what happened this morning. Would you mind sharing with me more?"

Assessment of morbid jealousy symptoms	I can imagine that you have gone through a very difficult period. Can you share with me when you started to suspect your wife is having an affair?	Can you describe your recent relationship with your wife? Is there any event that triggers off your suspicion? How did you arrive at the conclusion that your wife is unfaithful? Can you share with me your evidence? Do you know the identity of the third party? Do you follow your wife? If yes, how often? How often do you call your wife? Do you search her belongings (such as hand phone, text messages, underwear, handbag, and credit card bill?)	Could there be other possible explanations for her behaviour? If I give you a scale from 1–10, 1 means that you do not believe that your wife is unfaithful: How do you rate your belief? I can imagine that you have gone through a tough time. What is your plan for your marriage? Are you going to divorce your wife? Are you going to confront her? How do you cope with the current situation?
Risk assessment	Have you thought of harming yourself? If yes, how would you do it? What would you do to your wife if she denies the affair? Will you be more aggressive?	Are you going to take any action against the third party? If yes, how would you do it? Do you have any children? How old are they? What are their views on the current situation? Have you ever thought of harming them?	Do you have access to weapons? If yes, what kind of weapons do you have? Do you carry weapons with you? When will you use it?
Psychiatric comorbidity	Can you take me through how much you drink in a day? Has there been an increase in alcohol intake recently? Have you developed further problems as a result of drinking?	Do you encounter any sexual problem (such as inability to maintain erection during sex?) If yes, how long did you have this problem? Was it related to diabetes?	How is your mood at the moment? Do you feel sad? Can you tell me more about your sleep, appetite, and energy? How do you see your future? Do you feel guilty? How is your confidence level? Do you experience anxiety? Can you tell me more about your fear (such as losing your wife)?

	When people are stressed, they turn into recreational drugs. Have you tried those drugs?	Can you tell me more about your past relationship? Did you suspect your partners or girlfriends in the past? Have you been unfaithful to your partners in the past?	Do you have unusual experiences such as hearing voices when no one is around? Do the voices give instructions? Do you feel that someone wants to harm you at this moment? Do you think that there is a plot behind your wife's infidelity? How do other people describe you as a person? Do they say that you are more suspicious? Do you have problems with your friends or neighbours? Do you trust them?
Past history	Do you have any encounter with the police? If yes, for what reason? What was the consequence? Have you ever appeared in court? If yes, were you sentenced to the correctional service?	Can you tell me more about your diabetes? What kinds of medication do you take? Do you take them regularly? Have you ever experienced low sugar level and felt very giddy? Were you violent at that time?	

Common pitfall:

a. Failure to cover the range and depth of the information required for this station.

**Important to assess risk of harm to self, wife, the third party, and children.
Ascertain if the patient has any concrete plans and when he plans to do it.

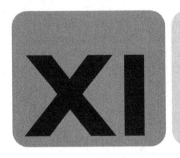

Information to candidates:

Name of patient: Mr Jenner

You have assessed Mr Jenner and determined that he is likely to have been suffering from a delusional disorder, that of morbid jealousy. Mrs Jenner is in the hospital, and she is hoping to speak to you as she wants to know what is wrong with her husband.

Task: Please speak to Mrs Jenner and explain to her regarding her husband's diagnosis as well as the appropriate management plans for him.

Outline of station:

You are the wife of Mr Jenner and are very concerned about his sudden outrage and aggression today. You're worried as you feel that he is not his normal self. You understand that the psychiatrist has seen him and would like to hear more about the diagnosis that the psychiatrist has given him. In addition, you wish to find out more about the management should he have an underlying psychiatric condition.

CASC Construct Table:

The CASC Construct Table is formatted such that candidates would be able to cover adequately both the range and depth of the assessment required in this station.

Starting off: "Hello, I am Dr Melvyn. I have just seen and assessed your husband. I understand that you have some concerns that you would like to discuss with me today. Can we have a chat?"			
Clarification of the diagnosis	I understand that this has been much of a surprise for you, and I understand how difficult you must have felt in that situation. I understand your concerns about your husband's condition. I have seen him and done the necessary assessment.	From what he has shared, he has a strong belief and conviction that you are having an extramarital affair. Are you all right with me going on? I have tried to challenge the beliefs that your husband has, but he remains strongly convicted.	He has a condition known as morbid jealousy, a subtype of a delusional disorder. Have you heard about this condition before? In such a condition, an individual usually has a firm and unshakable belief that is out of keeping with the cultural norms.

DOI: 10.1201/9781003313113-III

Clarification of risk issues	I am quite concerned about the risk issues that your husband possess. Throughout the conversation, he remains quite convinced of his beliefs. I am also concerned about your safety.	In addition, I also gathered that your husband has been using alcohol daily, which might predispose him to further violence. I understand that he does not have any previous convictions or forensic involvement. Is that true?	Given what has happened today, I will recommend that your husband be detained under the Mental Health Act for a period of treatment in view of him being unwell currently and the further risk he might pose.
Provide an overview of the management plans	I hear your concerns about the treatment options that he might be put through if he is detained. About treatment, there are available medications to help him with his condition.	When he is more stable, psychological treatment might be suitable to help him with his condition. The medications that we are considering for your husband are antipsychotics. These would help with the fixed convictions that he currently harbours against you.	As discussed, when he is more stable, we could try to engage him with psychological therapies or talking therapies. A common psychological therapy we routinely recommend to our patients is cognitive behavioural therapy. Do you have any questions about the management of your husband's condition on the ward?
Provide an overview of the longer-term management plans if he is discharged to the community	In the longer term, we need to consider gradual reintroduction of your husband back into the community. We could consider granting him Section 17 home leave when he is better and have a community nurse accompany him home.	You could tell us how his condition is, and we will discuss how best we can help your husband's condition with the rest of the multidisciplinary team members.	When he is eventually discharged home, we hope to be able to continue engaging him with our community mental health team. I know that I have provided you with quite a lot of information. Please let me know if you have any questions for me.

Common pitfall:

a. Failure to cover the range and depth of the information required for this station.

**In this station, the wife may be very insistent for the patient to be discharged. Therefore, it is important to highlight to her the high risk that he poses. Use patient's symptoms to highlight the characteristics of morbid jealousy. Explain to wife in layman terms what "delusion" means.

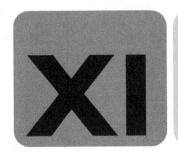

STATION 112
EROTOMANIA AND
STALKING BEHAVIOUR
(HISTORY TAKING)

Information to candidates:

Name of patient: Mr Wilson

You have been tasked to speak to Mr Wilson, who has turned up at the emergency department of one of the hospitals today looking for a nurse who treated him three weeks prior. He was arrested by the police as he wielded a knife against the security staff that prevented him from looking for the nurse.

Task: Please speak to the patient and elicit his abnormal beliefs. Please also conduct a detailed risk assessment.

Outline of station:

You are Mr Wilson and have just been arrested by the police. You merely turned up at the emergency department to look for the nurse—"Anna"—who treated you weeks ago. From your brief encounter with her, you strongly believe that she has given you cues that she is in love with you. You know some details about where she lives and her contact number. There was also an occasion during which you stalked her. However, you decided to look for her in the hospital's emergency department today as you knew that she would be on her shift.

You have made plans for tonight, including how you would want to engage her in intimacy. You were arrested when you wielded a knife at the security staff who tried to stop you from seeing her. This is not the first time you have gotten involved with the police. When you were with your previous girlfriend, something similar happened. You are not very willing to engage with the psychiatrist as you believe that the police have got the wrong person and that you have every right to see her. You are convinced that the nurse is in love with you.

CASC Construct Table:

The CASC Construct Table is formatted such that candidates would be able to cover adequately both the range and depth of the assessment required in this station.

DOI: 10.1201/9781003313113-112

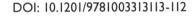

Starting off: "Hello, I am Dr Melvyn. I understand that you have been to the hospital today to look for one of the nurses, and the police have since arrested you. Can we have a chat?"			
Assess current behaviour	Can you tell me why you are under police custody at this moment? What is your relationship with the nurse? What have you done to her thus far? Do you know her name? How do you feel towards her?	How much do you know about her? Do you know her number? If you do, how often do you call upon her? Would you resort to leaving a voice message if she does not respond to your call? Do you mind telling me the contents of your voice message? Do you happen to know where she lives? How did you find this out?	Why do you need to take these actions? Do you want to be close to her? From your view, how does your behaviour affect her daily life?
Risk assessment	Are you planning to do anything to the nurse? If so, would you mind telling me the details? Do you plan to harm her? If yes, what would you do? Is this part of the fantasy?	Have you ever applied force on her? What was her reaction? Did she defend herself? Would you do it again in the future?	Have you thought of harming yourself? (or) Are you so stressed with your current situation that you have had thoughts of ending your life? Has anyone tried to stop you from following her? If yes, what did you do? Do you carry a weapon? Will you use it to harm others who try to stop you?
Differentiation between types of stalker	**Incompetent stalker** Did you encounter any difficulty having a relationship in the past? Does the nurse remind you of the unpleasant past? **Rejected stalker** When you are ignored or rejected by the nurse, how do you feel? Do you feel that both of you were in a relationship? Do you hope to reconcile by following her?	**Intimacy seekers and erotomania** Are you in love with her? Do you think she is in love with you? Do you think she will love you? How certain are you that she is in love with you? Can it be a misunderstanding? Do you have sexual feelings towards her? **Resentful stalkers** Have you tried to frighten her? Are you taking revenge on her?	You have followed her a lot. Do you feel stressed? Do you want to continue this behaviour? Have you thought of changing yourself? Do you think you need treatment?

(Continued)

(Continued)

Forensic and psychiatric history	Did you have trouble with the police in the past? If yes, what was the reason? Were you charged subsequently? Did you break any court orders in the past? Have you seen a psychiatrist in the past?	How often do you drink? What kind of alcohol do you drink? What would you do if you were drunk? Do you also use any recreational drugs?	

Common pitfall:

a. Failure to cover the range and depth of the information required for this station.

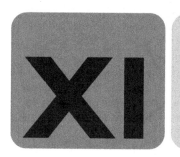

Information to candidates:

Name of patient: Mr Wilson

You have been tasked to speak to the nurse, Anna. She understands that you have since assessed the patient (who was the one who turned up to look for her). She wants to find out more information. She wants to know the risks involved and what she ought to do.

Task: Please speak to Anna and explain to her the current situation. In addition, please inform her about the relevant risks involved and address all her concerns and expectations.

Outline of station:

You are Anna, a senior nurse working in the emergency department of a local hospital. You were told by the management that there was a man who turned up at the emergency department today and requested to speak to you. He claimed that you knew him. You have treated many patients over the course of the past few weeks and have no recollection of who this patient is. You were told by the management that the patient has informed them that he strongly wishes to see you as he believes that you're in love with him. You were told that, when he was prevented from seeing you, he wielded a knife at the security staff. The police were called in, and he was subsequently arrested. You understand that the psychiatrist has since seen him. However, you also learned from the management and the police that he was subsequently released by mistake and is currently in the community. You're worried about the associated risks. You wish to know what precautions you ought to be taking.

CASC Construct Table:

The CASC Construct Table is formatted such that candidates would be able to cover adequately both the range and depth of the assessment required in this station.

DOI: 10.1201/9781003313113-113

Starting off: "Hello, I am Dr Melvyn. I understand that you have heard about what happened this morning. I understand that you do have some concerns. Can we have a chat?"			
Explain assessment	I understand that it must have been very distressing for you. I assessed the patient before he was released. I hope that I can share my assessment. I hear your concerns about you not knowing him. I have spoken to him at length. I must break confidentiality and share some of my assessments with you.	He did share with me that he received treatment from you a few weeks ago, when he was in the observation ward for panic symptoms. From that meeting, he strongly believes that you're in love with him. I do understand that you would have treated him just like any other patient.	During my assessment, I attempted to challenge those beliefs that he has. These beliefs that he has are quite fixed and cannot be challenged. My assessment is that he might suffer from a delusion of love, or "erotomania." Have you heard about this before? This is a condition in which the individual has a firm belief that others are in love with them. The belief is typically firmly held and not challengeable.
Explain the associated risks involved	I hear your concerns with regards to the fact that he is currently out in the community. I'm sorry to hear about this. I believe the police are doing their best to try and locate him based on the information they have about him.	When I spoke to him, he shared with me some other information, which I think you need to be aware of. I'm quite concerned about the risk he might pose to you. During the assessment, he did share that he knows where you stay and also that he has your contact number. In addition, he claimed that there was an occasion in which he stalked and followed you home.	Moreover, during the assessment, he also shared that he does have sexual fantasies about you, and he desires for intimacy with you. Is it all right for me to go on?

Address concerns—immediate plans for the nurse	I know that you're deeply concerned about the risk he poses. We are also deeply concerned about your safety.	Given that he knows where you live and has your contact number, I do not advise you to head home for the time being. Do you have friends or family with whom you could potentially stay with? Thanks for sharing with me your alternative accommodation plans. I understand you are quite concerned about leaving the hospital and getting to your accommodation. We will speak to the management as well as the police, who could potentially provide you with some assistance in the meantime.	I will also inform the management about my assessment briefly and advise them that they allow you to go on a short period of leave as it would be dangerous for you to return to work currently. Do these plans sound reasonable for you? Are there other concerns that you have now?
Address concerns—management plans for the patient	We will advise the police to continue their search for him. If the police manage to find him, he is likely to be detained for further assessment.	Should there be a need, we might need to apply the Mental Health Act to detain him for further assessment and treatment.	Please be assured that he will not likely be detained in the hospital you work in, in view of the current risks posed.
Provide reassurance	Thanks for speaking to me, and I hope that I have addressed all your concerns and expectations.	I know that you are deeply troubled by the current situation, but we will work jointly with you, the management, the police to ensure your safety.	Do you have any other concerns that you would like to raise?

Common pitfall:

a. Failure to cover the range and depth of the information required for this station.

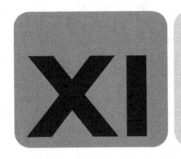

STATION 114
VIOLENCE RISK
ASSESSMENT
(MSE EVALUATION)

Information to candidates:

Name of patient: Mr Ward

You have been tasked to speak to a 32-year-old male, Mr Ward. He was arrested by the police and transferred to the emergency department for further evaluation. He was arrested because he broke into the house of his ex-girlfriend. He has a known history of schizophrenia and underlying antisocial personality disorder and was released from the prison eight months ago.

Task: Please speak to him and perform a mental state examination. Please also attempt to perform a comprehensive risk assessment.

Outline of station:

You are Mr Ward and have just been arrested by the police. You were caught for breaking into the house of your ex-girlfriend. You were released from prison around eight months ago. You were previously arrested and convicted for housebreaking as well. Since your release, you have not been taking the medication that was prescribed for you whilst you were in prison. Recently, you started to experience auditory hallucinations as well as paranoia. You decided to break into your ex-girlfriend's house as you believe that she is part of this plot in which others are against you.

CASC Construct Table:

The CASC Construct Table is formatted such that candidates would be able to cover adequately both the range and depth of the assessment required in this station.

DOI: 10.1201/9781003313113-114

Starting off: "Hello, I am Dr Melvyn. I understand that you have just been arrested by the police. Can we have a chat so that I can understand how best I can help you?"			
Explore circumstances of the current offence	I received some limited information from the police regarding what has happened today. Would you be able to tell me more?	Thanks for sharing. Did you make any plans prior to your current attempt? What plans did you make? Can you tell me how you managed to break into the house? What intentions did you have?	Did you drink any alcohol before your attempt? Did you use any substance before your current act?
Explore MSE—delusions	Can you tell me more about why you feel this way? Can there be any other alternative explanations for this?	Do you feel that other people are trying to harm you in any way? Do you feel that other people are talking about you?	Do you feel that you have some special powers or abilities? Do you feel that certain things have special meaning for you?
Explore MSE— hallucinations	**Auditory hallucinations** Do you hear sounds or voices that others do not hear? How many voices can you hear? Are they as clear as our current conversation? What do they say?	**Second-person auditory hallucinations** Do they speak directly to you? Can you give me some examples of what they have been saying to you? **Third-person auditory hallucinations** Do they refer to you as he or she, or in the third person? Do they comment on your actions? Do they give you orders or commands as to what to do? Are you able to resist them?	How do you feel when you hear them? Can there be any alternative explanation for these experiences that you have been having?
Explore MSE— thought disorders	**Thought interference** Do you feel that your thoughts are being interfered with? Who do you think is doing this?	**Thought insertion** Do you have thoughts in your head that you feel are not your own? Where do you think these thoughts come from?	**Thought broadcasting** Do you feel that your thoughts are being broadcasted, such that others would know what you are thinking? **Thought withdrawal** Do you feel that your thoughts are being taken away from your head by some external force?

(Continued)

(Continued)

Explore MSE— passivity experiences	Do you feel in control of your actions and emotions?	Do you feel that someone or something is trying to control you?	Who or what do you think this would be?
Risk assessment and insight	With all these troubling experiences, have you thought of ending your life?	Have you thought of taking revenge on the people you think are troubling you?	Can you share with me your plans (should you have any)? Do you have access to any weapons?
Assessment of anti-social personality disorder	Have you been involved with the police before? Can you tell me more? Have you ever stalked anyone before? Have you ever lied or deceived others? Have you been involved in any fights with others? Have you assaulted others?	With regards to your prior offences, do you feel remorseful of what you have done? How do you feel towards the victim?	How would you describe yourself in your personality? Do you feel that you could be impulsive in your actions at times?
Personal history	I understand that you have previously seen a psychiatrist. Do you know what diagnosis the psychiatrist has given you? Do you know the rationale for you to be on medication? Do you have family members who have mental health–related issues as well?	Do you drink? If you drink, how often do you drink and how much? Do you use any other illicit substances?	Thanks for speaking to me today.

Common pitfall:

a. Failure to cover the range and depth of the information required for this station.

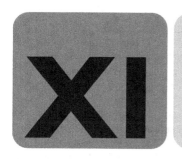

STATION 115
VIOLENCE RISK ASSESSMENT (DISCUSSION AND MANAGEMENT)

Information to candidates:

Name of patient: Mr Ward

You have been tasked to speak to a 32-year-old male, Mr Ward. He was arrested by the police and transferred to the emergency department for further evaluation. He was arrested because he broke into the house of his ex-girlfriend. He has a known history of schizophrenia and underlying antisocial personality disorder and was released from the prison eight months ago. You have been tasked to speak to the consultant, Dr Richards, to discuss further about your assessment.

Task: Please speak to the consultant and discuss the management plans for this case.

Outline of station:

You are Dr Richards, the psychiatrist in charge of the inpatient unit. The nurse manager has informed you about this case, and you wish to find out more information to determine if the patient needs further inpatient management.

CASC Construct Table:

The CASC Construct Table is formatted such that candidates would be able to cover adequately both the range and depth of the assessment required in this station.

Starting off: "Hello, I am Melvyn. I would like to discuss with you the case which I have just assessed in the emergency department."			
Explain events leading to admission	Based on the history shared by the patient, he claimed that he planned for the housebreaking today. He claimed that his thoughts were no longer within his control, and he suspects his ex-girlfriend is involved in a plot to harm him.	He wanted to break into the house to get back his belongings, as well as to leave a message to threaten the victim. He denied harbouring any homicidal ideations of harming others.	He was arrested today for housebreaking, as he was spotted by others in the area.

(Continued)

(Continued)

Summarize mental state observation	I have briefly assessed his mental state. He has overt paranoid ideations towards others, as he has been thinking that others around him are intending to harm him.	In addition, for the past month, he reports that he has been increasingly bothered by auditory hallucinations. He also reports that he does not feel in control of his actions.	He has quite limited insight into his existing mental health condition. However, he recalls that he has been diagnosed with schizophrenia and has been on medication whilst he was previously convicted. He claimed that he has since recovered from his previous episode of schizophrenia. He mentions that he is no longer keen to be on medication.
Discuss risk assessment	I have done a risk assessment, as well, in view of the current circumstances leading to the admission.	The patient denies harbouring ideations to harm others. In addition, he denies harbouring any ideations to harm himself. Also, he was not intoxicated nor was he using any drugs when he attempted the housebreaking.	However, he was recently released from prison for a similar offence. He has no other history of any violent behaviours.
Explain management approach	Given his poor insight and his current risk assessment, I would like to recommend that he be admitted for further stabilization in the inpatient unit.	There is a high risk of him not being compliant with the recommended treatment if we were to engage him as an outpatient. We could potentially reconsider the introduction of antipsychotics for him and consider other strategies to ensure his compliance.	When he is more settled inpatient and is due for discharge, we could consider engaging him with the community psychiatric nurse to reinforce his compliance to medication, as well as monitor his mental state.

Common pitfall:

a. Failure to cover the range and depth of the information required for this station.

**In this station, you will need to stratify the patient's risk of violence and highlight the risk factors. It would be impressive if you could also mention what are some of the questionnaire tools you can use to assess violence risk, e.g. HCR-20 and the Psychopathy Checklist-Revised (PCL-R).

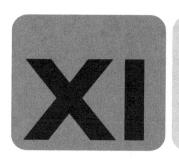

STATION 116
SEXUAL OFFENCE
ASSESSMENT

Information to candidates:

Name of patient: Mr Evans

You have been tasked to assess Mr Evans. He was brought in by the police for an assessment as there is an allegation that he has been sexually inappropriate with a child. The police are awaiting your assessment before they proceed with the necessary charges against him.

Task: Please speak to Mr Evans and explore more about the circumstances of the alleged offence. Please take an appropriate history to come to a diagnosis.

Outline of station:

You are Mr Evans and have just been arrested for an alleged sexual offence. You know that you are due to see the psychiatrist for an assessment. You are aware that your neighbour has called upon the police with regards to the alleged offence. You know the victim and have been taking care of the victim on several occasions. When questioned about the alleged offence, all you will share is that you were playing a game with the victim, and he accidentally brushed himself against your groin area. You will be cooperative otherwise and will share more about your psychosexual history. You are married, but you are not in a good relationship with your wife. Otherwise, you will deny any interest in pornography and other sex materials. You have received a previous warning for a similar offence.

CASC Construct Table:

The CASC Construct Table is formatted such that candidates would be able to cover adequately both the range and depth of the assessment required in this station.

DOI: 10.1201/9781003313113-116

Starting off: "Hello, I am Dr Melvyn. I'm sorry to hear that the police have arrested you today. Can we have a chat about it?"			
Elicit circumstances leading to current arrest	I'm sorry to hear that the police have arrested you. Are you aware of the reasons for the current arrest? Given the nature of the allegations, I do need to ask you some personal questions. Would that be all right with you?	Can you describe to me what actually happened today? Can you tell me more about your relationship with the victim? How long have you known him or her for? Can you share with me how frequent you have cared for the child?	Would you mind telling me more about where you were when the incident happened? Was there anyone present at that moment? I received news that the allegation involved you being intimate with the child. Can you tell me more?
Explore patient's view about alleged offence	Thanks for sharing with me the account of what has happened. You mentioned that the child brushed against you. What happened after that?	Did you get sexually aroused when that happened? I'm sorry but I do need to ask you some personal questions. Did you feel sexually aroused when that happened today? If you did, what did you do thereafter? Did you have an erection? Did you masturbate thereafter?	Given the current allegation made against you, how do you feel currently about all that has happened today? Very often, we do come across news about sexual offenders. What is your view on that?
Explore psychosexual history	Are you currently in any relationship? Can I know how long you have been married? Can you tell me more about how your relationship with your wife has been? I'm sorry to hear that you have been having some difficulties with your relationship currently.	Before being married, were you in any other relationships? Can you tell me more about those past relationships? Do you remember what age you achieved puberty? Do you remember at what age you had your first masturbation? Would you mind sharing with me more about your intimacy? At what age did you first have an intimate experience with a partner?	Sometimes, when people are having difficulties with the sexual side of their relationship, they turn to other materials to fulfil their needs. Do you watch pornography to satisfy your desires? Can you tell me more? Have you ever engaged in any other behaviours to achieve sexual arousal? Do you find yourself particularly attracted to children?
Explore the psychiatric and forensic history	Have you seen a psychiatrist before? Is there any history of any mental health disorders in your family?	Have you been involved with the police or the legal system before? Can you tell me more?	For the previous offence, what was the charge? Can you share with me what happened thereafter? Currently, are you in contact with any children?

Common pitfall:

    a. Failure to cover the range and depth of the information required for this station.

**It is important to remain empathic towards the patient and not appear judgemental.

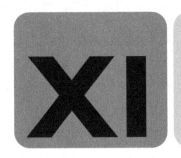

STATION 117
FITNESS TO PLEAD
ASSESSMENT

Information to candidates:

Name of patient: Mr Burton

You have been tasked to speak to Mr Burton. He was just arrested by the police following a shop theft at the local store. Whilst he was in the remand cell, he vocalized to the police officers that he has been on regular follow-up with the local mental health service and has been on psychotropic medication.

Task: Please speak to Mr Burton and explore more about the circumstances leading to the current offence. Please perform a brief mental state examination and assess whether he is currently fit to plead.

Outline of station:

You are Mr Burton. You have been arrested for your involvement in a shop theft. You told the police that you have been on regular psychotropic medication and have been on regular follow-up with the local mental health service. They have since referred you for further assessment. You have residual auditory hallucinations, but otherwise, you do not have any first rank symptoms. You carefully planned for the current offence by making sure that you stored items in an area that was not covered by the CCTV. You do understand the current charges pressed against you and do understand the differences between pleading guilty and not guilty. You have a basic understanding of the court proceedings as you have been to the court just six months ago for the same offence.

CASC Construct Table:

The CASC Construct Table is formatted such that candidates would be able to cover adequately both the range and depth of the assessment required in this station.

DOI: 10.1201/9781003313113-117

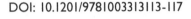

Starting off: "Hello, I am Dr Melvyn. I'm sorry to hear that the police have arrested you today. Can you have a chat about it?"

Explore circumstances leading to the current arrest	Thank you for speaking to me today. Can you tell what happened?		
Explore MSE—delusions	Can you tell me more as to why you feel this way? Could there be any alternative explanations for this?	Do you feel that other people are trying to harm you in any way? Do you feel that other people are talking about you?	Do you feel that you have some special powers or abilities? Do you feel that certain things have special meaning for you?
Explore MSE— hallucinations	Auditory hallucinations Do you hear sounds or voices that others do not hear? How many voices can you hear? Are they as clear as our current conversation? What do they say?	Second-person auditory hallucinations Do they speak directly to you? Can you give me some examples of what they have been saying to you? Third-person auditory hallucinations Do they refer to you as "he" or "she," in the third person? Do they comment on your actions? Do they give your orders or commands as to what to do?	How do you feel when you hear them? Could there be any alternative explanation for these experiences that you have been having?
Explore MSE— thought disorders	Thought interference Do you feel that your thoughts are being interfered with? Who do you think is doing this?	Thought insertion Do you have thoughts in your head that you feel are not your own? Where do you think these thoughts come from?	Thought broadcasting Do you feel that your thoughts are being broadcasted, such that others would know what you are thinking? Thought withdrawal Do you feel that your thoughts are being taken away from your head by some external force?
Explore MSE— passivity experiences	Do you feel in control of your own actions and emotions?	Do you feel that someone or something is trying to control you?	Who or what do you think this would be?

(Continued)

(Continued)

Explore fitness to plead	Can you tell me more about what the police are intending to charge you for? What do you think are the possible consequences?	Can you tell me your understanding regarding "pleading guilty"? Can you tell me your understanding regarding "pleading not guilty"?	Have you been in court before? Do you know the people who will be there? Can you tell me more? Do you know the process of the court hearing? Do you have a legal counsel who is representing you? Do you know how to instruct the lawyer to represent you? Thanks for sharing with me.

Common pitfall:

a. Failure to cover the range and depth of the information required for this station.

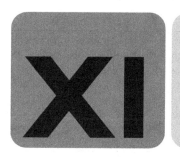

STATION 118
EXHIBITIONISM
(HISTORY TAKING)

Information to candidates:

Name of patient: Mr Bailey

You have been tasked to assess Mr Bailey. He was brought into the emergency room after he was arrested by the police for exposing himself in public.

Task: Please speak to Mr Bailey and obtain a history to establish a clinical diagnosis. His wife is here as well and has indicated her desire to speak to you in the next station.

Outline of station:

You are Mr Bailey and have just been arrested by the police. The police have arrested you as your neighbour has lodged a police report after she witnessed you exposing yourself in the garden. You are angry at your neighbour for making the police report. You deny feeling any sexual arousal during the incident. You are willing to cooperate much later into the interview and will answer the questions posed by the psychiatrist accordingly.

CASC Construct Table:

The CASC Construct Table is formatted such that candidates would be able to cover adequately both the range and depth of the assessment required in this station.

Starting off: "Hello, I am Dr Melvyn. I have received some information about what has happened. Can we have a chat about it?"			
Explore history of current presentation	Thanks for agreeing to speak to me. I have received some information about what has happened that led to your current situation. For me to help you, I would need to ask you some other questions. Would that be all right with you?	Can you tell me more details with regard to what has happened today? Can you tell me what you were doing when the incident took place?	Were you aware that your neighbour might be there? Has something similar to this happened before?

(Continued)

(*Continued*)

Explore patient's attitude towards current presentation	I'm sorry but I do have to ask you some personal questions. I hope you can answer them accordingly. How do you feel about the entire incident?	Due to the ongoing police investigations about you having exposed yourself, I need to ask if you felt any pleasure/arousal when you exposed yourself?	In addition, did you have an erection during the incident? On reflecting back on what happened, do you feel sorry for the victim? Do you feel guilty for your actions?
Explore psychosexual and forensic history	Can you tell me more about your relationships? Are you currently married? How long have you been married for? Do you have children?	How is your relationship with your wife? Have there been any difficulties with your relationship with your wife? Have there been any difficulties with the sexual side of your relationship with your wife? Do you have any other relationship before you got married? Can you tell me more about those relationships? Do you remember the first time you were sexually active? Do you remember when you first masturbated?	Pardon me for asking, but I would like to understand whether you have been previously involved with the police. Can you tell me more about what happened previously? Did the police charge you for the offence? What happened after that?
Explore psychiatry history and current mental state	Can I check whether you have seen a psychiatrist before? Is there anyone in the family who has a history of a mental health–related disorder? Do you use alcohol or any other substances? Can you tell me more?	Over the past month, how has your mood been for you? Do you find yourself having interest in things that you previously used to enjoy? Are there any difficulties with your sleep or appetite? Have you have had any unusual experiences? By that I mean, do you hear voices or see anything unusual when you are alone?	Do you feel that there are others out there who are trying to harm you? Do you feel in control of your thought processes? Do you feel in control of your emotions and actions?

Explore other possible diagnoses— cognitive decline and dementia	How has your memory been recently? Do you find yourself having difficulties remembering appointments or important tasks? Any accompanying physical symptoms (e.g. urinary incontinence, gait instability)? Any head injury or trauma?	Have others around you commented about your memory? How about others commenting about your change in personality?	Do you find yourself having difficulties with your daily activities? Do you find yourself having difficulties with your finances? Is there anything else you wish to share with me?

Common pitfall:

a. Failure to cover the range and depth of the information required for this station.

**In the case of an elderly patient, you need to assess whether there is any cognitive impairment that may affect his judgment and impulse control. In a younger person, you would want to rule out any organic brain syndrome.

**Differential diagnosis in this case includes paraphilia, psychosis, dementia, organic brain syndrome, and being under the influence of psychoactive substances.

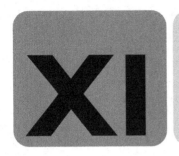

Information to candidates:

Name of patient: Mrs Bailey

You have already assessed Mr Bailey following his arrest by the police after he exposed himself in his garden. His wife is here, and she is keen to find out more from you with regards to your assessment. She has some concerns that she would like to clarify with you.

Task: Please speak to Mrs Bailey—"Sarah"—and address all her concerns and expectations.

Outline of station:

You are Mrs Bailey and are very concerned about your husband's condition. You are concerned as this is not the first time this has happened. In the past year or so, this has happened at least thrice. There was another occasion last month when your husband nearly exposed himself in front of your grandchildren. You are very concerned about the safety of your grandchildren as they do come over regularly over the weekend. You are extremely worried about the confidentiality of the information shared and want the core trainee to reassure you that all the information shared will be confidential. You do not want your grandchildren to be taken away or your access to your children to be restricted. If the core trainee explains that there are times in which confidentiality needs to be broken, you will appear to be extremely upset and low in your mood. You would like to understand from the core trainee what form of help might be available for your husband. You then share with the core trainee that you have been feeling low in your mood in view of your husband's condition. You do have most of the clinical symptoms of depression, and the core trainee needs to ask you about these symptoms in the consult.

CASC Construct Table:

The CASC Construct Table is formatted such that candidates would be able to cover adequately both the range and depth of the assessment required in this station.

DOI: 10.1201/9781003313113-119

Starting off: "Hello, I am Dr Melvyn. I have just spoken to your husband. I understand that you have some concerns about his current condition and the situation that has happened today. Can we have a chat?"			
Explain assessment	I'm sorry to learn of all that has happened to your husband today. I have seen him just now and done an assessment of his condition.	He denies that he has exposed himself intentionally. He denies any active psychiatric symptoms currently.	However, I'd like to check with you more about his condition. Were you present when the incident took place? Can you tell me more about what happened? Have you noticed any recent changes in your husband? Has there been a change in his mood or his personality? How has his memory been?
Explore risks	Thanks for sharing with me. I understand that it has been a difficult time for you. Prior to the incident today, can I check whether your husband has been involved in similar incidents previously?	Can you tell me more? Do you remember how frequently these incidents happen?	Were the police involved? Did the police press charges against him?
Dealing with confidentiality	It seems to me that you have some information that you wish to share. The information that you share will be kept confidential and is important for us in helping your husband with his current condition.	I'm very concerned to hear that there was an episode in which your husband nearly exposed himself to your grandchildren. I'm sorry but this involves a risk to a third party, in this case, your grandchildren.	It is thus essential for me to break confidentiality given the nature of the information shared as it would involve a risk to your grandchildren. We might need to inform the child protection services. I'm very sorry to be having to inform you about this.

(Continued)

(Continued)

Explain possible investigations, assessment, and treatment	It sounds to me that your husband has been experiencing significant memory difficulties for the past year or so. One of my considerations for his current condition might be that of dementia.	I would need to speak to him again to gather more information. The information that you provided me with regard to his memory difficulties is helpful as well.	We would also need to run some baseline blood investigations and probably also organize a baseline scan of his brain. This would help us in establishing the diagnosis. We might also recommend that he undergo further cognitive testing and maybe a neuropsychological battery of tests. If he does have dementia, there are a variety of options which we could recommend in terms of how best we could help him with his current condition.
Picking up on possible depressive symptoms in the carer	How have you been coping thus far? It seems to me that you are quite affected by all that has happened. How has your mood been for you?	Do you find yourself having interest in the things that you used to enjoy? How has your sleep been for you? What about your appetite?	Apart from this, are there other stressors in your life? Have you ever felt that life is hopeless and no longer worth living? I understand that you are in a difficult position currently in view of the ongoing issues involving your husband and the potential risks he poses to your grandchildren.

Common pitfall:

a. Failure to cover the range and depth of the information required for this station.

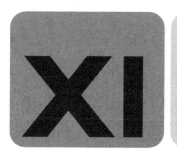

In this station, candidates are typically asked to assess for a variety of extrapyramidal side effects. The common side effects include (a) pseudo-parkinsonism, (b) acute dystonia, (c) akathisia, and (d) tardive dyskinesia.

The following lists some of the recommended steps:

- Seek consent from the patient before starting the examination.
- Ask the patient whether he has any pain in any particular region of his body.
- Make use of the alcohol rub prior to commencing the examination.
- Allow the patient to be seated down for the examination.
- Inform the patient that the examination involves an examination of his mouth, getting him to move his upper and lower limbs, and getting him to walk.
- Start the examination by observing the patient at rest.
- Observe for any movement abnormalities in his limbs and trunk.
- Ask the patient if he has anything in his mouth before getting him to open his mouth. In the event that he is wearing dentures, please get the patient to remove them. You will have to ask the patient to open his mouth twice. It would be best if you observe whether there are any abnormal movements of his mouth at rest. Subsequently, you need to ask the patient to repeat the steps again, but this time, with him sticking out his tongue. Again, please observe for any abnormalities of his tongue.
- Examine the patient's upper extremities for Parkinsonism-like features. Observe whether the patient has any baseline tremors by getting him to hold both his arms in front of him. Next, proceed to manipulate his arms and check for both lead-pipe rigidity as well as cog-wheeling. Ask the patient to gently tap his thumb with each of his fingers and observe whether he appears to have any difficulties with these movements.
- Ask the patient to sit at rest and observe whether he has any abnormal bodily movements. Get the patient to place both his arms in between his legs and observe once again for any abnormal movements.
- Ask the patient to stand up and get him to walk. While you are with the patient and he is walking, please observe his gait. Also, take note of whether he has reduced arm swing.

DOI: 10.1201/9781003313113-120

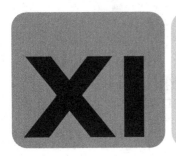
The following lists some of the recommended steps:

- Seek consent from the patient before starting any examination.
- Ask the patient whether he has pain in any region of his body.
- Make use of the alcohol rub prior to commencing the examination.
- Ensure that a chair is available for the patient to be seated at. Seek consent and ensure that the neck is adequately exposed.
- Begin by inspecting the neck, checking for any apparent goitres or swellings. Also, check for the presence of any previous surgical scars. Concurrently, also inspect the facial features for any signs of hyper- or hypo-thyroidism.
- Make sure that there is some water already available. Ask the patient to take a sip of the water and swallow. Inspect to see if the swelling rises on swallowing. This might suggest that the swelling is either a goitre or a thyroglossal cyst.
- Ask the patient to stick out his tongue. If it is a thyroglossal cyst, the swelling will move up.
- Proceed to palpation of the lump but do remember to check in with the patient if he is experiencing any pain. Examine the site of the lump, size, and whether the lump is single or multiple. Ask the patient to swallow and attempt to see if you could get under the lump. Examine the surrounding lymph nodes and check for any enlarged lymph nodes. Also palpate the tracheal position and check for any signs of tracheal deviation.
- Next, attempt to percussed the sternum, checking for any dullness, which is indicative of a retrosternal extension of the goitre.
- Attempt to auscultate the goitre then to check for any bruit.
- If time permits, please examine the eyes and check for reflexes.

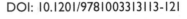
DOI: 10.1201/9781003313113-121

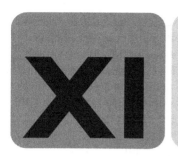

- Introduce yourself to the patient and seek consent for the examination.
- Ask the patient if he experiences any pain in any areas of his body.
- Make use of the alcohol rub before commencing the examination.
- Ensure that the patient's arms are adequately exposed before commencing the examination. For female patients, please ask for a chaperone. Should an examination couch be available, the patient could be positioned to be sitting on the side of the examination couch.
- Start off with an inspection of the patient's upper limb. Check whether there are any surgical scars or any wasting of the muscles. Inspect to check for any involuntary movements of the muscles. Inspect to determine any abnormal movements, such as chorea, myoclonus, or pseudo athetosis.
- After inspection, ask the patient to hold their arms out in front of them, with their palms facing upwards, and look for signs of any pronator drift. Please observe for at least 20 seconds. It might be helpful to ask the patient to also close their eyes to better observe for pronator drift.
- The next step of the examination involves an examination of the muscular tone. You could do this by asking the patient for his permission to hold onto their hand and elbow, then asking them to relax and gently move all the muscles of the shoulder, elbow, and wrist through their entire full range of movement. By doing so, observe whether there is an increase in tone, such as the presence of any rigidity and cogwheeling (which are signs associated with parkinsonism) or a decrease in tone.
- The next step of the examination involves an examination of the overall power of the upper limbs. Please examine the following: shoulder abduction, shoulder adduction, elbow flexion, elbow extension, wrist extension, wrist flexion, finger extension, finger abduction, thumb abduction. Please grade the muscle power using the MRC scale.
- Next, proceed to examine the reflexes. It is important to explain to the patient how you will be attempting to do this. Please also ensure that the upper limb is entirely relaxed before examination. Examine the biceps reflex, triceps reflex, and the supinator reflex.
- Check and examine sensations to light touch, pinprick, and vibration. Please be sure that you compare both sides during each of the examinations.

- Lastly, test for coordination to check for the presence of any cerebellar signs. To perform the finger-to-nose test, make sure that your finger is positioned in such a way that the patient has to reach out their arms fully to reach your finger. Inform the patient to touch their nose using their index finger, and then to touch your fingertip. Instruct them to do this as fast as they could. To check for dysdiadochokinesia using the pronation/supination upper limb test, ask the patient to tap the palm of one hand with the fingers of the other rapidly for a few times, and then rapidly switch hands.
- Thank the patient for cooperating with you on the examination and summarizing the main findings.

- Introduce yourself to the patient and seek consent for the examination.
- Ask the patient if he experiences any pain in any areas of his body.
- Make use of the alcohol rub before commencing on the examination.
- Ensure that the lower limbs are adequately exposed, but while doing so, ensure the modesty of the patient. For female patients, please ask for a chaperone.
- Start off with an inspection of the patient's lower limbs. Check whether there are any surgical scars or any wasting of any muscles. Look out for any obvious joint pathologies or any joint malformations. Observe the posture of the limb.
- Inform the patient that you need to palpate their limbs. Palpate the temperature of both sides of the lower limbs and measure the limb girth.
- The next step of the examination involves an examination of the overall power of the lower limbs. Please grade the muscle power using the MRC scale. Ask the patient to lift the leg up and try to resist against you. Then ask the patient to bend their knee and resist your attempt at straightening it. Then ask the patient to attempt to straight their leg while you are resisting against it. Next, ask the patient to bend their foot up and attempt to push the examiner's hand away. Ask the patient to step down and attempt to push the examiner's hand away. Lastly, ask the patient to point their toes up towards the ceiling against resistance.
- Test next for the following reflexes—knee, ankle, and plantar reflex.
- Ask the patient to stand up and walk. Observe the gait to check for any involuntary movements. Ask the patient to then place their feet together, keeping their arms by the side, and closing their eyes (Romberg's test). Stand near the patient so that you can stop the patient from falling over during this test.
- Test for sensation if there is time. Test for superficial sensation, vibration sense, and positional sense.

DOI: 10.1201/9781003313113-123

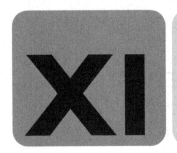

- Introduce yourself to the patient and seek consent for the examination.
- Ask the patient if he experiences any pain in any areas of his body.
- Make use of the alcohol rub before commencing the examination. For female patients, please ask for a chaperone.
- Cranial Nerve 1: Ask the patient whether he can smell (some sample of coffee which is provided).
- Cranial Nerve 2: Inform the patient that you are going to test his eyesight. Make use of a Snellen's chart to test the patient's visual acuity. In the process of testing, ask the patient to close one eye and test each eye individually.
To map out the visual fields, position yourself opposite the patient. Ask the patient to look straight ahead and cover their right eye with their right hand. Begin to move your fingers from the upper visual fields and then slowly in towards the centre of the visual fields, asking them to inform you as soon as they can see your finger. Repeat from the upper right, then upper left, then lower right and lower left of the visual field, and then repeat for the other eye. Perform a fundoscopy if one is available. Inform the patient that you will be shining a light into their eyes and that it may be uncomfortable when testing for their pupillary light reflex. Inform them to see at a distant target. While they are doing so, shine a pen torch into each eye and observe for a direct and consensual light reflex. To test accommodation reflex, inform the patient to look at your finger (which is positioned at a distance), and then bring your finger to within 10 cm of the patient, and look at the pupils to check whether they converge equally.
- Cranial Nerves 3, 4, 6: To test for these cranial nerves, position the patient in front of you, and inform him that he has to look ahead, directly into the eyes of the examiner. Ask him to follow the movement of your finger. You should describe the letter *H* using your fingers. Check for any abnormal movements of the eyes.

DOI: 10.1201/9781003313113-124
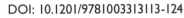

- Cranial Nerve 5: To test out the sensory component of this cranial nerve, inform the patient that you will be using cotton wool to gently dap on both sides of his face, in the location of the three main dermatomes. Remember to alternate between the different sides of the face. When doing so, ask the patient to tell you if he is able to feel the cotton wool. To test out the motor component of the cranial nerve 5, ask the patient to perform the following series of actions: (a) clench their teeth as tightly as possible, and you should be able to palpate the masseters and the temporalis; (b) ask the patient to attempt to open his jaw against the resistance of your hands.
- Cranial Nerve 7: Ask the patient to attempt to close his eyes as tightly as possible. You should then attempt to open their eyes.
- Cranial Nerve 8: Before testing, please check whether they have any pre-existing hearing impairments. Position yourself at least 60 cm away from the patient and whisper a number or word. Then ask the patient to repeat the word/number back to you. Assess both ears. If a tuning fork is available, advise the patient that you need to perform additional tests, namely a Rinne test and a Weber test, if there is time at the end of the entire assessment.
- Cranial Nerves 9 and 10: Ask the patient to open their mouth and make the sound "ah." Observe to see if the uvula is central and observe the movements of the soft palate.
- Cranial Nerve 11: Position yourself behind the patient and ask the patient to shrug their shoulders while you apply some resistance. Next, ask the patient to turn their chin against your hand in both directions, and at the same time, feel for the action of the sternomastoid muscle.
- Cranial Nerve 12: To assess this, instruct the patient to open their mouth, with their tongue within. Do a general inspection of the tongue, to see if there is any evidence of any wasting or any forms of involuntary movements. Next, ask the patient to stick the tongue out and move it from side to side and also to press their tongue against their cheek.
- Thank the patient before ending the examination. Inform the patient of any relevant findings.

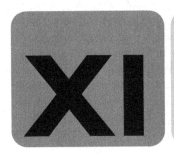

- Introduce yourself to the patient and seek consent for the examination.
- Ask the patient if he or she experience any pain in any areas of his or her body.
- Make use of the alcohol rub before commencing the examination. For female patients, please ask for a chaperone.
- Start off with a general examination of the patient. Look at their hands, and check their nails for signs of any pallor, clubbing, or cyanosis. Check also for splinter haemorrhages. Observe for the presence of any palmar erythema. Palpate the pulse and observe the rate and rhythm. Check both sides to determine if there is any radio-radial delay.
- Examine the eyes and the faces. Check the eyes for the presence of any jaundice or pallor. Look for any xanthelasma.
- Palpate the carotids by checking it one at a time. When doing so, also check the JVP. This could be done by asking the patient to lie down on a couch, while maintaining a position at 45 degrees. Ask the patient to turn his or her head to one side and inspect the height of the JVP.
- Proceed next with the examination of the chest. Inspect to determine if there is any obvious deformity, any visible pulsations, and the presence of any scars. Next, attempt to locate the apex beat, and do an assessment of the nature of the thrust. When examining the chest, also examine for the presence of any thrills.
- Next, make sure to perform auscultation of the following areas: mitral, tricuspid, pulmonary, aortic.
- Offer to take the patient's blood pressure if a blood pressure monitor is available.
- Examine the abdomen to check whether there are signs of any hepatomegaly or splenomegaly.
- Also check the legs for the presence of any peripheral oedema.
- Thank the patient before ending the examination and inform the patient/ examiner of any relevant findings.

DOI: 10.1201/9781003313113-125

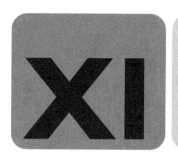

- Introduce yourself to the patient and seek consent for the examination.
- Ask the patient if they experiences any pain in any areas of their body.
- Make use of the alcohol rub before commencing the examination. For female patients, please ask for a chaperone.
- Assessment of gait: Ask the patient to walk towards the end of the room, turn, and walk back towards you. When doing so, please observe the gait of the patient. An ataxic gait is suggestive of an underlying cerebellar aetiology.
- Next, ask the patient to walk with the heels to their toes towards the end of the examination room.
- Next, perform Romberg's test. Ask the patient to place both feet together, and keep their arms by their side, and close their eyes. Stand close to the patient so that you can catch them in case they fall over.
- Perform the heel-shin test by asking the patient to slide a heel down from the opposite knee.
- Check for nystagmus of the eyes. This could be done by asking the patient to look straight ahead and asking them to use their eyes to follow your finger (use your finger and move it in an H pattern). Check for the presence of any abnormal movements of the eyes.
- Perform the finger-to-nose test. Ask the patient to reach out their arm, and to make use of the tip of their index fingers to touch your fingertip. Vary the position of your fingertip and ask the patient to continue to use their fingers to touch your fingertip.
- To check for dysdiadochokinesia using the pronation/supination upper limb test, ask the patient to tap the palm of one hand with the fingers of the other rapidly for a few times, and then rapidly switch hands.
- Thank the patient before ending the examination and inform the patient/examiner of any relevant findings.

DOI: 10.1201/9781003313113-126

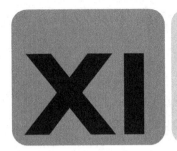

- Introduce yourself to the patient and seek consent for the examination.
- Ask the patient if they experience any pain in any areas of their body.
- Make use of the alcohol rub before commencing the examination. For female patients, please ask for a chaperone.
- Explain to the patient that the examination involves shining a light source into the patient's eyes, and it might be uncomfortable.
- Perform a general inspection of the patient's eyes to check whether there is any obvious redness, swelling, or discharge from the eyes.
- Have the patient seated and darken the examination room.
- Ask the patient to look straight ahead for the entire duration of the examination.
- Check for the presence of a fundal reflex—this is done by shining a light towards the patient's eyes and checking to see if there is light being reflected back from the retina.
- Adjust the ophthalmoscope settings, taking into consideration any corrections that need to be made in view of your/the patient's reflective errors.
- When using the ophthalmoscope, ensure that you approach the patient at an angle of 10–15 degrees. Make sure that if you are assessing the patient's left eye, you are holding the scope on your left hand. Attempt to visualize the disc by identifying a blood vessel and following the blood vessel to the optic disc. When the optic disc has been identified, assess the colour, its margins, the cup, and the diameter.
- Next, ensure that you assess each of the individual quadrant of the retina.
- Ask the patient to look directly at the light and inspect the macula (this is usually located laterally to the optic disc and appears yellow in colour).
- Repeat the previous steps for the other eye.
- Thank the patient before ending the examination and inform the patient/examiner of any relevant findings.

DOI: 10.1201/9781003313113-127

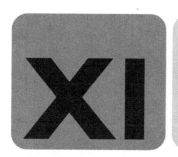

- Introduce yourself to the patient/examiner.
- Check that the patient's name and date of birth on the ECG are correct.
- Check the recorded date and time when the ECG was carried out.
- Begin by computing the heart rate. This is computed by counting the number of large squares between two consecutive QRS complexes, or between two consecutive R waves (the R-R interval), and then dividing 300 by this number of large squares. Normal rate is between 60 to 100 beats per minute.
- Comment on whether the rhythm is normal. A normal rhythm allows for the visualization of a P wave.
- It is important to remember that the P waves are representative of atrial systole and the QRS complex ventricular systole. T waves indicate ventricular relaxation.
- To determine if the heart rhythm is regular or irregular, locate the positions of three successive R waves, and check that all the intervals are the same.
- Next, determine the axis. A normal axis is observed if the QRS complex in leads I and II are mostly positive. If only lead I is positive, but leads II and aVF are negative, then this signifies the presence of left axis deviation. If lead I is negative, and leads II and aVF are positive, this indicates a right axis deviation.
- Examine the ST segment to determine if it is flat (normal).
- Check the QT interval. The corrected QT interval can be computed using the Bazett formula: QTc = (QT interval)/(square root of the RR interval). It should be less than 0.42 seconds.

DOI: 10.1201/9781003313113-128

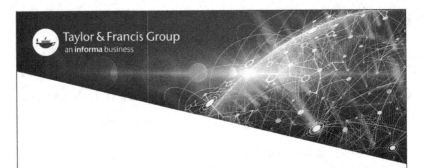

Printed in the United States
by Baker & Taylor Publisher Services